I0471190

GETTING OUT FROM THE FUNHOUSE TUNNEL

How I overcame Superior Oblique Myokymia

Second Edition

by

Simon Beider

Getting out from the funhouse tunnel
Copyright © 2013, 2014 by Simon Beider.

Printed version

ISBN-13: **978-1492113935** (CreateSpace-Assigned)
ISBN-10: **149211393X**

Classification

Library of Congress: **RE91-912**
Dewey: **617.762**

SOMer by SOMpeople® SOMpeople® by the Owner/Administrator of the online support group "**superiorobliquemyokymia.yuku.com**".

Chapter IX. Vision As A Metaphor, is a contribution of Sir Martin Brofman, based on his article "Vision as a Metaphor", reproduced with permission. Copyright © 1990 by Martin Brofman. Founder of the Brofman Foundation for the Advancement of Healing.

Chapter X. Exploring The Mind/Body Connection To Vision, is a contribution of Sharukh Vazifdar based on the article "A return to vision" reproduced with permission. Copyright © 2000-2013 Life Positive Foundation.

Chapter XI. Can Our Eyes Heal Naturally, is a contribution of Martin Sussman based on the article "Releasing The Inner Barriers To Seeing: Exploring The Mind/Body Connection To Vision!" Reproduced with permission. Copyright © 2009 by Martin Sussman. President and Founder of the Cambridge Institute for Better Vision.

Chapter XIII. Stress Management, is a contribution of Helpguide.org © Helpguide.org. All rights reserved.

Picture 9: Eye of God. NGC 7293: The Helix Nebula. Credit: NASA, WIYN, NOAO, ESA, Hubble Helix Nebula Team, M. Meixner (STScI), & T. A. Rector (NRAO).

All other trademarks are the property of their respective owners. The author is not associated with any product or vendor mentioned in this book.

DEDICATION

To my children, for pulling me out from the funhouse tunnel, and to those people with whom I did not have to pretend that everything was "just fine".

SIMON BEIDER

CONTENTS

SIMON BEIDER

SIMON BEIDER

ACKNOWLEDGMENTS

I would like to express my greatest gratitude to the people who have helped and supported me, both throughout my SOM experience, as well as this project.

María: I can't thank you enough for your thoughtful advice, and true understanding, from the beginning, up to this day.

A special thank of mine goes to my friends, whom I did not have to tell a thing, to notice I was going through difficult circumstances.

I am grateful to those who knew, and told me on my face some truths I had to hear.

To those who knew, and supported me listening in silence.

As well as to those that did not know, but I am sure that if they did, they would have stood by me.

I want to thank those who kept by my side at the moment of highest distress. I am so sorry for the fears and worries I could bring to you.

I want to express my gratitude and give credit to the founders and fellow SOMers at SOMpeople®, the online support group for people with SOM, for the initiative creating this group and the courage of sharing their experiences.

It is a privilege that Martin Brofman, Martin Sussman and Sharukh Vazifdar generously were willing to enrich this book with their bright insights, and Helpguide.org with its crystal-clear and practical information.

My appreciation to Tammy, for letting the cover of this book shine out with a striking design.

At last, but not the least; to my wife, for her stubbornness to stand by me in spite of my imperfections.

Thank you all, since you did not have to see to believe.

DISCLAIMER

This information is not presented by a medical practitioner and is for educational, informational, encouraging and motivational purposes only. The content is not intended to be a substitute for professional medical advice, diagnosis, or treatment. Always seek the advice of your physician or other qualified health care provider with any questions you may have about a medical condition. Never disregard professional medical advice or delay in seeking it because of something you have read. This book is not aimed to diagnose, treat, cure or prevent any disease. Nothing on this book should be understood as an attempt to offer or provide medical opinions or the use of traditional or alternative medicine.

INTRODUCTION

"The health of the eye seems to demand a horizon. We are never tired, as long as we can see far enough." - Ralph Waldo Emerson

* * *

I have never thought I would write this book.

In fact, I was writing other two related to my profession when I suddenly realized that it would be more useful, sharing my experience on SOM (Superior Oblique Myokymia).

Corporations can wait a few months; people do not. I always wanted to write a book, I left all others aside to get this done.

I am not a Medical Doctor nor an eye-care practitioner. I am only a person that got SOM and wants to help others.

This book is not a scientific paper. It is solely based on empirical knowledge and thorough documentation of my own journey.

I would have been so happy, if I had had the analytical sensitivity and sharper thinking required to interpret and understand all what was going at that time.

Unfortunately, I had to walk all the way one step at a time. There are no shortcuts for this learning.

I am going to share with you, my own experience, fully comprehensible only in retrospect.

I summed it up and wrote it in English, although it is my second language. I did it in spite of any grammar mistake I could have made (for which I hope you excuse me in advance), but I wrote it in English for your own convenience and accessibility.

I honestly do not know if this book has any literary merit. Not that I care that much, though. That is not the reason why I am writing this book.

I am definitely aware I am not Dan Brown, this book is perfectible in every aspect, except on the fact that it is really honest and perfect in intention.

The truth is that I am really fine, and I have left behind SOM as I knew it. Every experience of success that we dare to share is another rung up on the same ladder we all were forced to climb.

When my SOM started, I needed to read something like this so badly, I prioritized time over writing excellence and content over form.

I do not want this book to add a dose of stultification to SOM because of its medical nature. I kept my writing fresh, plain and jargon-free.

This is a modest book. It is the book I needed to write to confer my SOM journey a higher meaning and bring it to a proper end.

For you, this book hopefully will deliver what you are expecting for and need to know.

To let go this sharp experience, I had to share its learning. Realize, release and reveal it; that is –to me- the end-to-end course of this journey. And this is that last stage of the sequence.

This book was meant to help. I want this book help those who suffer from SOM, their relatives, friends, colleagues and everyone who want to know, not what SOM is, but rather HOW is to live with it.

Essentially, this book aims to reach those who have SOM. For you, the first and most important thing I want to tell you, is what I would have liked to hear years ago:

I DO UNDERSTAND YOU.

SOM is frustrating. It could unquestionably become a handicap ailment, which is only understood by the beholders and seldom observable by others.

I hope this book may carry you through your SOM experience. Notice that, in this case, I am using the word "experience" instead of "condition", to highlight the fact that you can overcome this challenge.

In any case, I hope that my experience will encourage you to ask all the questions you may have to the proper professional.

Ask your doctor about anything you may read, and eventually put this book on the test and consider what worked out for me.

If you are reading this book because someone you care is affected with SOM, I hope you can see how it challenges him or her, and from this information you may find a way to provide some aid, support and cheer.

I want this book reach eye-care professionals, as a resource to get their patients' viewpoint, serving to establish a more trustworthy relationship between patients and doctors.

Hopefully, this experience of mine will drive to findings that shine light on a barely discussed topic that help alleviate this unacknowledged condition, which – as far as I know- has not been thrashed out very well.

In order to do so, I was pondering a lot about how to deliver this work, deciding that you should feel free to copy, distribute and transfer it (if necessary).

I just would like to know if this effort succeeded reaching all the people that could need it, whether they can afford it or not.

Please follow the ripple effect of kindness. Share this book if it is needed, and if it is possible, let me know your kind review at Amazon.com.

That will be my reward.

At the beginning

I began writing this book with some concern which –of course- raised with the time (it could not have been any other way).

My first concern was that, because of the personal nature of the content, whether I should use a pen-name or not. Could it undermine the honest nature of this book? I have nothing to hide, but I have found a lot of bias towards people with sight problems.

I do not want to be stigmatized by SOM, but I am not willing to stop helping those who may need the lessons I have learned from it.

The second fear was related to the effects of writing. It has been such a long time since I am fine and SOMless, I was worry that writing about my experience would be like invoking some spell which might prompt SOM again.

At a point, I reproached myself to get exposed to such an endeavor which I knew it would mean a setback.

I was afraid to open de Pandora's box. It may seem harmless, but what if that turns out to have serious and far-reaching consequences? What if, recalling my experience, spend a lot of time in front of the screen or writing triggers my SOM again?

Many months ago and after all I went through, my closest circle was angry with me for absorbing the stress of writing this book, not to mention that when they found out I was doing it in a second language, and that extra pressure I imposed upon myself, they simply wanted to lynch me.

But, the further along I get in writing this book, the more confident I became, and I enjoyed this endeavor, keeping in mind what I would have liked to read a few years ago when SOM was nothing but anxiety and uncertainty.

Conventions used in this book

I used some words, which represents SOM-related concepts that you will find all along this book.

I found it practical, funny and helpful to keep in mind that this book is not intended to be a medical essay.

These are the silly conventions for our common convenience:

* ExercEyes: bodily activity that enhances wellness of your eyes and reduce SOM symptoms.

* EyeMotion: positive or negative mental state or mood, caused by or shown through the eyes.

* SOM: Superior Oblique Myokymia

* SOMbie: A person who has SOM.

* SOMday: A day with SOM symptoms. (It could be a nice SOMday or a hard SOMday).

* SOMer: A person who has SOM.

* SOMfriendly: A condition or property particularly suitable or beneficial for a person who has SOM.

* SOMless: Free from SOM symptoms.

* SOMtime: A moment or incident with SOM symptoms.

* SOMfree: A situation or condition free from SOM symptoms.

* Twitcher: A person who has SOM.

What you will find on this second edition

As a SOMer writer, the first edition was a fantastic experience. A lot of fellow SOMers got the book and eventually reached me asking further questions, or to provide some feedback.

I have taken note of those enquiries and comments and reviewed this book according.

I know you have high expectations, and I want to let you know in advance, what are you going to get from this book.

I do not want you to wander all along these pages in search of the key answers to SOM, so I added at the very beginning, a shortcut right to the "vital few", the essential frequent asked questions.

I am not saving the best for last, quite the reverse: I am letting you go straight to the burning issues. Isn't it fair? I think it is.

In this edition, this book is organized in four parts.

The first section is about how people with SOM see and interact with the world in each dimension of their life.

It begins with a series of examples of how cultural elements have been setting the visual system as the predominant psychological, cognitive and, social instrument.

Then, I share and let you know my own experience, which will let you get a comprehensive understanding about how SOM crumbles the quality of life. There are many tips that I applied myself, to mitigate the symptoms.

The second section is about the learning of this experience.

Along the text, you will find several pictures. Most of them are photos taken by me, modified to look as I actually perceived those moments.

There, you will find a deep understanding about the source of the condition, and a holistic approach to cope and overcome SOM.

In the third section, I share a few alternative vision about the meaning of SOM and some tips about how to deal with it.

Just for the record: the learning from this experience did not rely on metaphysical nor superstitious thinking. I will tell you about rough things such medication, therapy and other solid science resources.

However, fair is fair, you are going to find some alternative approaches that I have found along the way that –somehow- resonated with me, helping me to connect some dots and understand SOM with a universal approach.

I invited or quote some people that offer this viewpoint, just as extra tools instrumental to claim your quality of life back.

Like anything on this book, what I have found along the way, I bring it here. You can take it, or leave it.

At last, I share with you a wrap-up, with some conclusions, suggestions, lessons learned and an update about what has happened over the past 12 months.

SHORTCUT TO THE ESSENTIAL

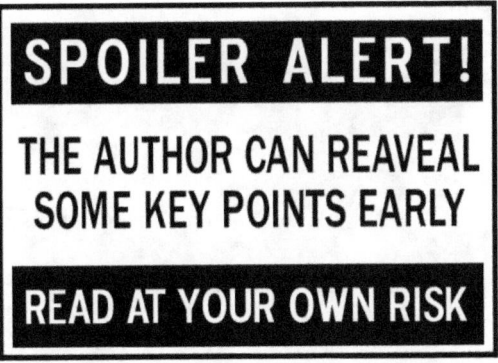

These are the most FAQ (Frequent Asked Questions) of the first edition's readers.

Please remember that I am not a medical doctor and the provided answers are based on empirical experiences:

1. Am I alone? Are there a lot of people with SOM?

You are certainly not alone. Nobody knows for sure how many people suffer from SOM, since it is a rare condition and there are no statistics or whatsoever.

I can tell you, though, that the first edition of this book was downloaded nearly 500 times, and it would be judicious assuming that they are fellow SOMers.

Based on downloads statistics and the people that reached me out, I drew a map where you can see that you may find people with your very same condition –at least- in the United States, Canada, Mexico, Argentina, Uruguay, United Kingdom, France, Germany, India and Japan.

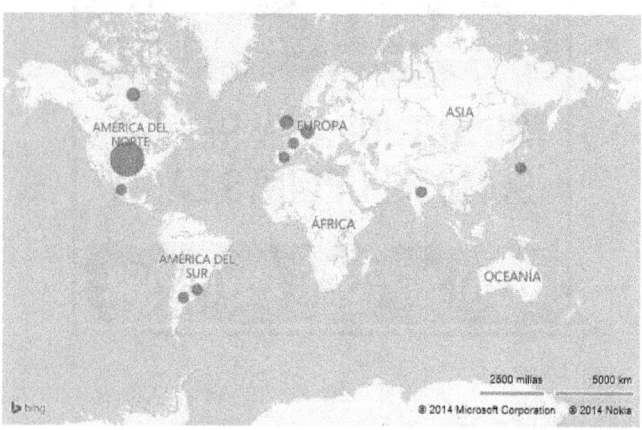

Picture 1: First edition's readers. Sorry the continents names are in Spanish.

2. Is SOM a severe disorder?

SOM is a non-life-threatening condition. It is not an

acute disorder by itself, but is as harsh as the symptoms you may experience.

Some people have just slight, sporadic and brief discomfort events on their eye sight, meanwhile others may suffer for constant and throbbing experiences with secondary effects.

3. Is it getting worse?

SOM is non-progressive, it is not contagious, will not produce further degeneration and it will not affect your "good" eye.

4. Is SOM curable?

Well, I would not dare to say it is curable, in terms that you can get rid of it for life, but it certainly is treatable and can become a chronic condition -as hypertension- that you can control.

SOM may be manageable through treatment, therapy, medications and surgery. You may also find alternative methods to get what it takes to gradually diminish its symptoms, enhancing your quality-of-life.

5. What kind treatment have your tried?

Oh gosh, I have tried almost everything, except invasive treatment such substance shots and surgery.

6. Did you try any medication?

Yes. I came across with an extraordinarily effective medication that should be prescribed by a professional.

7. Could you really get rid of SOM?

I got SOM curved until the point I have no symptoms at all, and if any, under very particular circumstances, its effects are so subtle and brief, that they are barely perceptible. And since I know what triggers SOM, I learned how to manage those factors, preventing SOM to occur.

8. What is the main trigger of SOM symptoms?

Stress.

9. Is SOM a handicap?

Sometimes. A disability is an impairment that substantially limits a person's capacity to perform life activities. A disability may include impairments that limit sight.

The term "disability" is used to qualify a person fairly for government benefits, special support, help or services.

All individuals with disability have impairment. However, a person can have impairment without disability.

For example, a person who wears glasses has

impairment, but does not have a disability; the impairment is correctable and therefore does not restrict performance.

However, a person declared legally blind is unable to perform certain functions, such as driving, and hence is said to have a disability that restricts performance.

In my experience, at certain point SOM was so brutal that —as it would happen with a person who is blind-prevented me from, for example, driving. I was just unable to do it.

So in order to be precise, I would say that SOM could be a serious vision impairment and eventually –if it absolutely prevents you from doing something relevant- it may become a handicap.

10. I take a glance at the book and I read some things, regarding Egypt symbols and Kabbalah stuff. Sorry, but I call bullsh*t on that.

That is OK. You are entitled to your own opinion. However you are misunderstanding the reason I included that text.

At some point of my experience, I wondered how come that I was so affected because of SOM, and I began to ponder and research about how our visual sense gained a dominance over others.

I refer to different sources and quoted several texts, providing examples of this idea, with the goal of trying to explain how, over the history, our culture was shaped, in a big extent, by a visual paradigm with symbols and stories related with the eye and sight.

Please, do not jump to the conclusion that I intended to assert that SOM is somehow related to Kabbalistic symbols or anything like that, that is not the point of the chapter.

At any rate, feel free to skip ahead all the philosophical issue, and go right to the following chapters. I promise, you are not going to lose any hands-on information concerning how to deal with SOM.

11. I read that you considered using a penname. Is Simon you real name? If not, why? Are you embarrassed of your SOM?

Simon is a penname, but I chose to use it not because I was embarrassed of SOM, but to prevent some bias at work.

I was afraid that people at work think I have a screw loose. SOM is related with "something linked to the brain" after all.

But it had a counter effect. After pretending for so long that there was nothing wrong, I developed tactics to disguise and mitigate SOM symptom that, although at some point effective, its outcome was a massive level of additional stress.

You know? I already felt overwhelmed, overloaded, unappreciated and with the dozen balls keeping in the air, and when I came across with SOM and the need of faking, I ended up burnout.

In order to make a long story short, I got fired, and the fear of being cast aside because of SOM continued.

A penname allowed me to write the whole experience without any kind of self-censorship and fear. Thus, I understood that a penname was necessary to keep the book as honest as it gets.

As Oscar Wilde said: "Give a man a mask and he'll tell you the truth".

Same thing.

12. Do you support the theory that you can fix whatever you want if you only have the right will, the right attitude and do it the right way. If you try it and it does not work, then you have only yourself to blame.

Not at all! I just mean that it happens that there is a common pattern among SOMer, which is that stress triggers SOM.

If you want to tame your SOM symptoms, chances are that you must learn about yourself. Meaning looking the patterns and association between the context, feelings, situations and when SOM is triggered.

In example: we all began thinking that there should be an object that triggers SOM, something such a carpet, or fluorescent lighting.

Well, perhaps it is not those stuff, but if the carpet and light belong to your workplace, chances are that the problem could be some psychological effect associated with your workplace or professional relationships.

In that sense, yes, you ought to have the courage (willing or attitude) to consider everything, and not to leave any factor behind.

If you are not willing to consider anything beyond objects and tangible substances as possible factors that may trigger your SOM, it is up to you, and nobody could judge you.

And if you tried to explore beyond, and it does not work. There is no reason to blame yourself nor anybody else.

13. Could anything good come out of SOM?

Yes. After your own journey, you could get to know yourself better. You could get more confident. You could learn how to decipher SOM symptoms as "warning notices" sent by your body. And you could appreciate some things that you used to take for granted.

14. Why did you write this book? Is this book for profit?

The only reason for writing this book, is to help others.

You'll see. At the beginning of my SOM experience I was afraid, lost and perplexed, and nobody could tell me anything about what was going on with me.

Looking back in time, I decided to put all the notes together (I took notes about everything I was experiencing) and write this book; the book I would have liked to read at that time.

This book is not for profit at all.

It is distributed via Amazon and its cost is the minimum that Amazon set to cover their own costs.

I also adhered to the lending program, so you can lend this book to another reader for up to 14 days.

One of the beauty of it, is that the borrower does not need to own a Kindle device and can read the book after downloading the free Kindle reading app.

Since this book is on the Kindle Owners' Lending Library, with Amazon Prime, you can borrow and read it on your Kindle device.

If you are subscribed to Kindle First you can borrow Kindle First books for free when they are released, so chances are that you will can read this book without any additional cost.

You can get this book internationally delivered for free via Amazon Whispernet.

In addition I took advantage of the Kindle Countdown Deals through which I am providing readers with limited-time discount promotions (available on Amazon.com and Amazon.co.uk).

Finally, the book owners could get the Kindle version of new editions at no cost.

All of these decisions, mean that I am doing everything to get no royalties or whatsoever.

15. I would like to thank you...

Well, a nice review at Amazon would be enough and very much appreciated, indeed.

PART I:
GETTING INTO
THE FUNHOUSE TUNNEL

CHAPTER 1.
THE TICKET FOR THE FUNHOUSE TUNNEL

"... I came to in the Crazy House, and for a while there, I thought it was me that was crazy. After what I would have been through, anything crazy at all seemed natural. But now I was sane..." Orson Wells. The Lady from Shanghai

* * *

Samuel Hahnemann a German physician, best known for creating the Homeopathy, once said "there are no diseases, but sick people".

As far as I know there are no two identical SOM experiences. Beyond common patterns, every patient is different and presents variations of the same disease.

But everyone could say that the worst thing about SOM, the worst thing that prevent you to get rid of it, is the fact that nobody can fully understand how it feels.

I was alone for years. I wish you find some comfort knowing that you are not alone, and someone else understands you.

I do know that after a certain period, dealing with tremors and uncontrolled movements of your eye you suddenly feel as going through a frightful funhouse tunnel… during an earthquake.

I have been there. I do understand you, and I am sure this fact certainly let you go half way out from the tunnel.

Everybody can google Superior Oblique Myokymia and eventually will find more than 11,700 results.

Any result describes, one way or another that it is an unusual chronic eye movement disorder where an eye muscle, the superior oblique, twitches periodically causing jumping of a single eye (Thurston and Saul 1991). SOM is probably caused by blood vessel compression of the trochlear (4th) nerve, at the root entry zone. (Hashimoto, Ohtsuka et al. 2004; Yousry, Dieterich et al. 2002).

Big deal! I am sure you already know that.

Googling further is pointless. You will only get pretty gory pictures of eye surgeries that will freak you out as they take you back to a scene from the Clockwork Orange.

It certainly does not help a bit.

The truth is that no one knows exactly what triggers it. There is no medical treatment or a silver bullet that resolves all the causes, stops or even lightens the symptoms, so it is in a great extend up to us –those who suffers it- responsible to find and exchange knowledge to find some relief.

Please, do not get me wrong: I know science can help, and it certainly defines the best it can what SOM is, but it needs time.

Yet, even if it gets to the point to be able to answer all the questions, it will not explain the anguish of living with it, nor the wounds it makes on your heart, mind and soul.

The first thing to realize is that, what affects the most, is not the twitch of the eye, but your own perception of yourself and your world.

As any other optical illusion, SOM does not work if you shut down your eyes. SOM may fool your eyes, but it aims to trick your mind.

You can choose to block your eyes, but that is not going to take you too far. You have to keep your eyes wide opened to preserve your peace of mind and keep it sharp to comprehend what lies beneath SOM.

Visual paradigm

The following paragraphs may sound a little odd, but summarize a concept I have been mulling over, during my SOM experience.

In a nutshell: we are visual creatures.

We live in a visual world. Our perceptions of the world, the information we capture and the signals we send, are awesomely visual in nature. Even our dreams are visual. We replay and re-create life visually in our minds. Even reading implies transforming the words into mental pictures.

Eyes are one of the most notable organs in earthlings, in fact, are the most complex one, after brain. Science says it took a few million years to evolve. On the other hand, some people claim to be an example of irreducible complexity, impossible to have evolved via natural selection.

One way or another, it is pretty obvious that one of the main physical characteristic that makes a modern human being is the fact to count on this remarkable visual capacity.

We live in a visual world, dominated by images on TV, in newspapers, magazines, movies and Internet.

This is only the beginning since media and technology bring, process and carry an overwhelming amount of information that is only possible to assimilate visually.

That is not news, ancient civilizations found them attached higher significances to the eye and vision.

Imagery of an all-seeing eye can be traced back to Egyptian mythology and the Eye of Horus.

Developed within the realm of Jewish thought, Kabbalah concept of the eye and its power is of major importance, as eyes are the only organ of human able to perceive the light (the abundance), and it does it expanding and contracting the pupil.

Kabbalist said that when you blink, is the only instant when your eye rest and can control how much light it gets. Like the pupil of the eye. The more light you shine on it, the more it will shrink.

When there is no abundance (darkness), the eye's pupil expanded as people should do spread themselves to capture as much positive energy as they can.

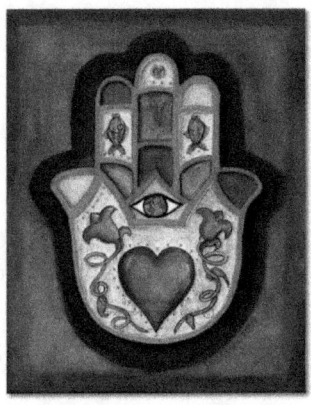

Picture 2: Hamza

The Hamza is a palm-shaped amulet popular throughout the Middle East and North Africa, and commonly used in jewelry depicting the open right hand, an image recognized and used as a sign of protection. The Hamza is believed to provide defense against the evil eye containing an eye symbol in the middle of the palm.

Just a trivial note: Hamza symbol has become a favorite among the world's most fortunate. Gwyneth Paltrow, Madonna, Naomi Campbell and Jennifer Aniston, among other Hollywood stars as and socialites, have begun wearing it.

The eye as a symbol also appears in Buddhism, where Buddha is also regularly referred to as the "Eye of the World" throughout Buddhist scriptures.

Caodaism **also** depicts the image of God **using the metaphor of the eye**.

The Bible begins with the Genesis, and almost every step of the Creation requested the conformity of God through His sight ("And God saw that it was good" or "pleasing to the eye" or "favor in the eyes of our lord").

There is surprisingly a unusually serious bias towards physical "imperfections" among those are some related to eyesight, such in Leviticus 21 when God present conditions to Aaron's descendants to get close to the altar:

"No man who has any defect may come near: no man who is blind (…) or who has any eye defect".

This is amazing, and I could not explain it, but based on the fact that, since Jewish people are the "people of the book", it is reasonable that in order to belong to the tribe, one should be able to read.

Joking aside, the Bible contains many stories that enforce the power of sight:

"There is no place God cannot see". "There is no situation He cannot discern". "He sees it all".

Scripture attests to this beautifully. Genesis 21:14-19 states the story of Hagar.

Abraham sent her off with her son. She went on her way and wandered in the Desert of Beersheba. When the water in the skin was gone, she put the boy under one of the bushes. Then she went off and sat down about a bowshot away, for she thought, "I cannot watch the boy die."

And as she sat there, she began to sob. (…) then God opened her eyes, and she saw a well of water. So she went and filled the skin with water and gave the boy a drink. What was the miracle? – Would ask the wise one It was not the spontaneous creation of a well of water, but that Hagar opened her eyes and could see the well.

* * *

"No object is mysterious. The mystery is your eye"
Elizabeth Bowen

* * *

According to the Gospel of Mark, when Jesus came to Bethsaida, he was asked to heal a blind man. Jesus took his patient out of town, put some spittle on his eyes, and laid hands on him.

"I see men like trees, walking," said the man. Jesus repeated the procedure, resulting in clear and perfect eyesight. "Neither go into the town," commanded Jesus, "nor tell anyone in the town."

Even though, early Christians would not have been happy that Jesus had to give two blessings to achieve a proper result.

In Medieval and Renaissance European iconography, the Eye of God (often with the addition of an enclosing equilateral triangle with a single eye inside it and almost always with rays emanating from it) symbolizes the omnipresence and omniscience of God, who watches over all things) was a clear image of the Christian Trinity.

Seventeenth-century depictions of the Eye of Providence sometimes show it surrounded by clouds or sunbursts. It is at the top of the Declaration of the Rights of Man and the Citizen, during the period of the French Revolution (on August 23rd, 1789).

It has been used as a symbol for many groups, associations, government agencies' shields and national flags.

Perhaps one of the best known of all can be seen on the reverse of every single one-dollar bill, the Great Seal of the United States topped by the Eye of Providence.

Even corporate logos such those of LucasArts, CBS, AOL, Endemol, NVidia, Time Warner Cable and Logitech, use the eye symbol.

There is no doubt the eye has been an influential and powerful image all over the world and along history.

As a derivate from the power of sight, it happened to acquire connotation of the highest order as divine conformity, social advantage, political control, moral and ethical leadership and cultural, intellectual, economic or ethnic superiority.

The simple capability to distinguish light from the darkness (as a metaphor of distinguish the good from the evil) through the sense of sight, is a power that seems to remain hidden in the roots of our culture.

Not to mention common phrases "Love at first sight", to express we feel instant attachment, "I see," to express we understand, and "Eyes are the windows of your soul."

The last phrase as the English proverb means the ability to join the world surround us with the inner being.

There are two quotes in the Bible that could be the root of this phrase:

Mark 7:20-23 states what could be the root of that quote: "The eyes are likened to the windows of the heart in." And Matthew 6:22 says "The lamp of the body is the eye."

The power of sight is unconditional and comprehends according to a person's inner will.

But at the same time looking in someone's eyes could decipher the nature of soul (or the strong emotions in our hearts).

If such a thing is true, what is the nature of the SOMer's soul that cause such a physical disorder?

How does it expose us? What reading other people may get through my SOM eyes?

There is nothing funny to be exposed in such a way, anyone could be able of reading my emotions; to "look into my soul" (metaphorically speaking).

It is not just the physical aspect of your life what is compromised. Whether you are aware or not, at a deep level, this "window" makes you feel vulnerable.

I know the above texts may sound weird, but the point is: How in the world we could be immune from such a strong cultural visual paradigm?

What is the connection between our vision, our eyesight, and our way of Being?

We all are deeply conditioned to think our eyes the main instruments to learn, live, survive, progress and transcend. Incidentally, the lack or damage of the visual sense means a significant weakness and a life-threatening disadvantage.

But that is just part of our belief system, just a set of reciprocally supportive views. The beliefs of any such system can be religious, philosophical, ideological or a combination of these.

Paraphrasing the British philosopher Stephen Law, belief systems are "claptrap" which can "draw people in and hold them captive, so they become willing slaves ... If you get sucked in, it can be extremely difficult to think your way clear again".

Helen's shining example

"He that has one eye is a prince among those that have none." Thomas Fuller

* * *

One of the most inspirational discovery during my journey, was "The Miracle Worker", the 1962 Oscar-winning feature film, starring Anne Bancroft and Patty

Duke, portraying the life of Helen Keller.

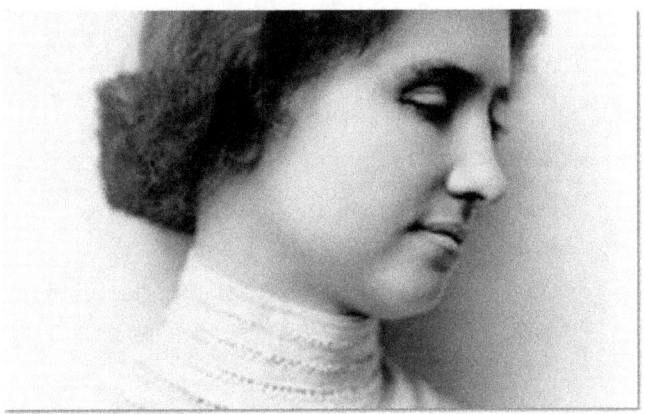

Picture 3: Helen Keller.

Helen was the first deaf-blind person to earn a Bachelor of Arts degree thanks to Anne Sullivan, her remarkable tutor, who got her rise above the seclusion, silence and darkness and a lack of language.

Think of it for a moment: a woman at the early days of the XX century that could overcome her condition, which inhibited her since the cradle, from the main sensorial instruments –sight and hearing- to discern, understand and interact with the world.

Finding her story was a remarkable coincidence (if such a thing exists). I found it just at the right time (or it found me).

How do my SOM may compare to Helen's adversities? How do I dare to think there is not a way to deal with it?

Knowing her struggle helped me to play down mine.

Before that, I thought SOM make a handicapped person out from me, but then I understand that I was wrong.

No matter the pain and the sadness and worries and frustration, there was a long way to get even close to that a real severe impairment condition.

If Helen overcame all the adversities of her fate, how could not I?

I was still able to interact with the world, enjoying the blessings offered by life, and making wonderful things during my existence.

Forget for a moment about what SOM prevent you to do.

As long as you still have a moment to grasp your children faces, to see your grand-daughter smile or contemplate a sunset, things are not that bad.

It is all about to make that remission last longer, making time itself, somehow, to be bend.

* * *

"Things seen are temporal, and things unseen are eternal" Helen Keller

* * *

Visual people

I realized that when the problem seems to be in your eye, the solution is in your brain.

Representational systems are a NLP (Neuro-Linguistic Programming) model that examines how the human mind processes information.

According to NLP most people use all of their senses but one system may dominate, even though the nature would be to get a dynamic balance based on the context and mood.

NLP asserts that three of the five sensory based modes dominate in our mental processing; they could be a combination of visual, auditory or kinesthetic.

I have always been eye-minded, with a strong tendency to visual thoughts. To me, since I was a kid, the conception of everything used to be almost exclusively based on the dominant visual sense, and consequently SOM affected me that much.

SOM could be particularly nasty for those who capture his perceptions and ideas of space through the sense of sight: visual people.

One of the most fascinating finding of NLP is that eye movements are indicators of cognitive processes.

Involuntary eye movements frequently come with thought processes, which access and use particular representational systems.

The American psychologist William James in his book Principles of Psychology (1890, pp. 193-195) observed that some eye micro movement always accompanies thought, what NLP calls "visual eye-accessing cue" (eyes moving up and to the left or right for visualization).

Later, psychologists such as Kinsbourne (1972), Kocel et al (1972) and Galin & Ornstein (1974) began to associate eye movements to brain processes.

They noticed that right-handed people tended to shift their heads and eyes to the right during rational and verbal tasks (left hemisphere), and to move their heads and eyes to the left during creative and spatially oriented tasks (right hemisphere).

That is people have a propensity to look in the opposite direction of the part of the brain they are applying to accomplish cognitive tasks.

Knowing this, I wondered if the SOM movements of my eye could be –somehow- related with emotion or thoughts.

I have tried to perform both intellectual and artistic tasks, in different environments, in order to realize which work and environment triggers SOM the most, and I did find a correlation of feelings and thought with SOMtimes.

Said that, I wondered what if SOM is not the cause of my feeling but the other way around.

Those who suffer SOM find that, no matter who you are, what you do and where you are, every aspect of our life is altered.

To set you free from the anguish, you have to express what you feel and do not pretend that everything is just fine.

Like diving or working at height, you need to go with the other person, to help you if you stumble along the way.

Therefore, we, the SOMers, SOMbies, Twitchers, should unlearn and throw off many labels and obsolete and mystical creeds.

Those ideas prevent people to consider the possibility to claim our quality of life back.

Blindness or vision problems do not hold anyone back from having a productive, active and exciting life.

You are entitled to demand an enjoyable life – NOW!

You have to be aware that it is up to you to understand, that if you want to get out from the funhouse tunnel, closing your eyes to avoid the situation is not the solution, but you have to move forward on the bridge walkway.

You have to keep in mind that even the most aggressive mind-blowing vortex attraction is effective, only if you can see at least a limelight.

You can still learn from even this awful ride, and once aware of it, you can put a stop to it and dismantled it for good.

If SOM bothers, at least it means that you are able to see, which is great, even though SOM tries to test your senses.

My great-great-grandfather left a diary with some notes and several peculiar quotes. One of them says: "I finally realized that, with health, I can heal myself of anything."

I found this diary during my SOM journey and this quote helped me realize, that as long as I could see, I could get better.

I hope you find it inspiring and encourages you to reach the handrails that allow you to pass through the tunnel.

CHAPTER 2.
PUSHED INTO THE FUNHOUSE
TUNNEL

When people ask me how did I overcome SOM, my immediate response is *"Per aspera ad astra"*, a Latin phrase which means "Through hardships to the stars".

As any other story, mine started several years ago, on an ordinary day, out of the blue and without any warning notice or of any kind.

It was like being pushed into a swimming pool, where I would have never been willing to jump; or even more precisely, it was like being forced to enter into a disturbing funhouse tunnel.

The first time I noticed that something weird was going on, I was at work. It suddenly got oddly hard to read on the screen. It was an unusual, subtle sensation which I was not able to distinguish.

I thought it could be eye strain (you know: fatigue, pain in and around the eyes, blurred vision and headache) that may take place after working and focusing on a computer monitor for a long time getting the eyes irritated and uncomfortable).

Then, I got out from the office to go to the restroom to wash my face, and refresh my eyes with cold water.

Once in the corridor, the whole hallway violently "rotated" around me about 30 degrees clockwise, to return in a blink to the original position.

Glassy eyed and perplexed, I stumbled and then I got up wondering "what the heck was that?!"

I thought it should be a consequence of the position of my neck looking down at the monitor placed a little lower than it should be, which forced me to adopt an awkwardly position causing, stiff neck or something.

A few weeks went by, hoping these episodes fade away, but they continued.

I went to the ophthalmologist. He suggested that it could be the CVS (Computer Vision Syndrome).

Back then I thought it was something associated to the working environment that exposed me to intensely bright overhead lighting, glare from the window walls and dirty vents of a brand new building where we recently got moved.

I knew that because the building was relatively new, the piping and vents were dirty because of the construction, and when they turned the air conditioner on, the dust in the air already have had caused a certain number of conjunctivitis.

But it was not what it seemed.

Even though I did not know it yet, I was being pushed right into the bridge walkway of the funhouse tunnel.

Just like gliding along a slippery slope, the symptoms began to rise, both in frequency, duration, and intensity, although they were difficult to describe.

I was scared and puzzled. I just did not know what was going on.

I had it the complete bundle of symptoms: neck pain, blurred vision, fatigue, eye strain, dry eyes, irritated eyes, double vision, and dizziness... everything you would not have wanted.

I remember paying a lot of attention at every symptom, trying very hard to understand them, as well as their causes and effects.

I used to run to the restroom to look at my eye on the mirror, trying to grasp something strange, but everything looked just fine, even if, at the same time, I was experiencing a bouncing vision.

Then I began to get seriously worry. I did not see anything anomalous on the mirror, so I thought the problem was into my head.

At home, I asked my wife to look at my eye and, with a mocking tone, she always had the same answer: "There is nothing wrong, don't worry."

I do not blame her. Nothing wrong was noticeable, and I have to admit it: I was "a little bit" hypochondriac... what the hell; the truth is that I used to be quite a good specimen!

I knew how it felt the anxiety and fear to get a serious illness based on a minor physical sign.

I was aware that from the external judgment, what I was saying, perfectly could have been another "false positive", another spin-off of the "Peter and the Wolf" tale, although I knew this was a brand new different story.

I was not even sure if the problem lied on one eye, both or into my brain.

Those whom I dare to mention about my experience, used to suggest it was eyelid twitching (the involuntary spasm of the eyelids muscle), but I had those in the past, and it was nothing like that.

However, since fatigue, stress, and caffeine triggers the eyelid twitching I wondered if the new experience shared the same triggers.

The SOM was getting acute.

I went to a new ophthalmologist and as soon as I told him my case, he jumped to the conclusion, that it was just a regular eyelet jerk.

He checked my eyes and did not find anything wrong.

I explained him, as good as I could, in many different ways, how I was seeing. Then he finally gave up, and said that the best thing to do was making an appointment with a neuro-ophthalmologist.

I dutifully did it at once, appointing me for the sooner available spot on the practitioner agenda.

A label at last

Quite excited, the practitioner addresses to his patient.

- "We already have your diagnostic: You have the Frankeheimer syndrome."

- "Is there a cure, doctor?"

- "We do not know yet, Mr. Frankeheimer."

* * *

Two weeks later, I was in the waiting hall.

By that time, I found something intriguing: moving my eyes to the bottom left corner, triggered some shakiness of my eye.

Although I hated it, I practiced it all the way to the doctor's office, and once there, I continued training the "trick" in the waiting room.

But Murphy's Law also applies to SOM, and during the eye examination, and during the test the corner trick mockingly did not work.

I tried harder. I moved my eyeball up and down, over and over again. My eye was like a yo-yo played by an extremely hesitant person. Nothing. "This b*tch is teasing me -I thought about my eye."

Note: on the first edition I was too shy and I omitted some bad language, but one reader asked me if I have been always impassive and if I ever swore because of SOM, and of course I did! So this edition is even more authentic (and less politically correct). I hope you do not mind.

I spent a great deal of time there. Eyeball up, eyeball down, eyeball to the right, eyeball to the left, chin over a machine that printed tickets with numbers, flashing light at my eyes, eye drops… I had it everything.

The practitioner was going to give up, and then he glimpsed a subtle activity on my right eye. "Gotcha! – He said- Wow! It is SOM".

He looked at me as I were a rare living specimen found in the Cryptozoology literature you know, the pseudoscience that searches for animals whose existence has not been proven such as Bigfoot and the Loch Ness Monster.

Well, I suddenly became the long-searched Yeti of the Ophthalmology.

-"Do you consume any drugs?" –he asked.

-"Only if chocolate and pizza apply" –I replied.

-"Did you hit your head with something?" –he asked. But I did not.

- "Have you been under stress?"

- "If I have been under stress? –I said. Doc, I live in Argentina! Just in the past decade I went through countless economic crisis. I lost my savings, my job, my family, my friends fled away; I hardly could pay the rent. As an individual I moved forward swimming upstream and professionally I felt like Indiana Jones making his way through the impenetrable jungles of Central America with a machete! Of course I have been under stress! As far as I concerned, my nationality is like a chronic disease! Not to mention I am having an awful time at work with rumors, intimidation, humiliation, discrediting and isolation. Stress is in my job description!"

This neuro-ophthalmologist –a maven on his field- was extremely professional and thoughtful. He thought me, in plain language, the known physical basis of SOM. In a nutshell: "uncontrollable random spasms of the muscle, the twitches, and the rotation of the eyeball" (which always reminds me the earth's rotation on its own axis).

"SOM". Then and there: the first time I heard of it. The problem was labeled, at last.

He acknowledged how little science knows about it and its triggers (except for the stress and stimulants such drugs, coffee, tea, etc. –that is why he asked about it before).

"It may leave as fast as it came." He said. "It can go tomorrow, next week, in a few months, a year… or ever".

"Great! –I thought- he is saying that SOM is not going to last forever, just until death shall tear us apart!"

How come that the improbable evil is easier to be accepted than the possible blessing?

"I will get rid of this thing! –I thought."

He told me I should not be afraid, but my condition was so rare, it was barely seen by any colleagues of him.

He told me that there are so few cases and so difficult to document, that the discipline knows about its existence, but does not go much further with reliable treatments or extensive understanding of my condition.

He told me that he was almost sure that it was SOM. How sure? Well, I should have an MRI to prove it was not a brain tumor or whatsoever.

And even it was not a tumor –the most terrifying diagnostic- It was an increasing tremor after all, and concerns went even further at a frantic fast pace:

Is it a progressive disease?

Is it life threatening?

Is it going to affect my vision forever?

Is it the first symptoms of Parkinson?

Is it hereditary? "Oh God, my children!" –I thought

Is it going to hit the "good" eye? – By the way: one eye was a living hell already both eyes would be a nightmare beyond description! The sole idea of having both eyes affected scared me to death.

The specialist answered all my questions as convincingly as it was possible, and mentioned some new procedures to put a stop to SOM.

He mentioned something about surgery, cutting or blocking a nerve or muscle.

Just thinking about it, crept me out. I couldn't even stand the TV series ER or Dr. House. I do not like seeing blood, specially mine!

Then he said something about a bizarre and unexplored Botox application.

Botox? That stuff based on the most acutely toxic substance? The life-threatening toxin that causes illness in humans and animals? Shut up near the optic nerve that goes right into my brain? And just to experiment?

"No way! -I thought."

I leave that to Hollywood stars. I could see myself looking fabulous and totally wrinkle-free, but speaking gibberish on a wheelchair!

"Sorry, I am not willing to go where no man has gone before". –I said.

So we agreed that I should go and return, based on how my SOM progress (even though "progress" is not the most suitable word to describe it).

Triggers

In order to find some way to reduce the symptoms, I had to check every possible element that set off SOM.

I wrote down every single factor and condition that I suspected could trigger my SOM episodes.

These are a few of my favorite things:

Environment: weather; air conditioner; heaters and ventilation; lighting; Pressure and humidity (very dry weather) and seasonal changes. This is a catch-22 because when the weather is hot I feel more comfortable indoor where air/conditioner is turned-on and when the weather is cold, and I am quite good outdoors, I find quite terrible with heaters or similar; fluorescent light; Sun glare; Heated, too dry or poor ventilated rooms. Helps a lot rooms with air conditioner or humidifier; carpet in the workplace; rubber flooring (like in exit stairways. Smell of glue + plastic); laminated plasticized wooden flooring (it began a few days after I plasticized the wooden floor at my place). Overcrowded places or events.

Physical conditions: Tiredness, insomnia, eye movements, conjunctivitis, allergies, stiff neck, headaches. Stress, fatigue, eyestrain (long day in front of the screen or extensive reading) or insufficient sleep.

Previous conditions and medicines: Astigmatism. Old glasses. Conjunctivitis. Allergies, sinus and/or upper respiratory conditions. Antihypertensive, Muscle relaxant.

Emotional conditions or situations: Stress, crisis, frustration and angry. Sudden unpleasant events and crisis. Mobbing (emotional abuse in the workplace).

Activities: working, long reading, taking notes, meetings. Looking down at a certain angle (after effects: stiff neck, headaches, etc.). When you work with a 22" screen, you move your eyes to the Windows "Start" button, and that is terrible. Had to get used to work with one eye shut. Sometimes it is an additional stress to pretend there is nothing wrong but the other party suddenly have 2 pairs of eyes, or you are presenting some slideshow, and you have to close your eye to target the right hyperlink (I hate that!). When eye contact is expected (I always paid attention to eye contact, and it was difficult to handle, but I manage it quite well even under this circumstances). Driving: depends on the environment. Air conditioner helps. To be placed under pressure or stress by constant solicitation.

Entertaining: movies, 3D and stage productions. (Especially with flashes and strobes).

Foods and drinks: coffee, tea or any infused drinks. Sugar consumption or excessive consumption of diet sodas.

Gadgets and technology: new 22" monitor, a new LCD TV set, Wi-Fi antennas or mobile antennas (you may laugh at me, it is not a conspiracy theory, but I felt SOM as an interference. I moved my Wi-Fi switcher. I never went as far as to considering on wearing a tinfoil hat to prevent some government from reading my mind though!).

Chemical exposure: cleaning products, insecticides. Smell of glue on plastic surfaces. Anti- deodorant or antiperspirant.

Cycle of Acceptance

You have probably heard about the stages of the Cycle of Acceptance: denial, anger, depression, bargaining and acceptance.

Not only that I went through all, but I even used to deal with all of them on a single day and even at the same time!

I was struggling with anger, depression and bargaining but, let's say, the center of gravity used to change depending on how hard SOM manifested itself during the day, which could shift drastically, from one day to other.

I could be complete hopeless one day, and hopeful the next one.

The very idea of "having a nice day" changed.

The simple question "how do you do?" prompted an endless chain of consideration; pondering a lot of factors related to my eye behavior, although the answer would have been a polite "fine, thanks".

"Fine?" Nothing like that! I was in constant pain, living in a constantly twitching and revolving world around me.

The more I tried to pretend that everything was just OK, internally fighting against the symptoms, all got worse.

I returned to the optometrist convinced that bright light triggered the eye jerking.

The only thing he found was that –at ironically as it may sound- my visual acuity (unaided) had improved since the last time I checked it, when I got my previous eyeglasses to adjust a subtle astigmatism.

I asked him to prescribe those Transitions lenses glasses that change shading depending on the light. Later on I found that what made them change was UV light; they do not change inside the car or at the office.

I was pretty sure bright light hurt me, and at some extent these glasses helped.

But it could be a double-edged sword: the gradual change of shade got me dizzy.

At my job, the office had an open layout. No walls at all, and fluorescent lights all over the ceiling.

At that time I considered having photophobia.

I tried to hide myself from bright lights, so I asked to move my place to the darkest corner of the office. I did not mind if I had to work into the maintenance closet.

After a year of wrestling against SOM, I went back to the first ophthalmologist.

Life with SOM sucked.

"Tell me what in the world should I do, please –I begged." And the man peacefully said something I will never forget:

"Look Simon, it happen that I am baldheaded, and you have a jumping eye. I had to get used to live with baldness; learn to live with your twitching eye".

It was one of those "A-ha" moments.

His advice was both funny, pathetic and yet exceptionally effective. It was far the best thing he could have ever said, and perhaps I could ever hear. A stunning waking call to go on with my life.

Against my professional instinct which is to find the source of the problems, I had to render it up.

If I had to live with SOM, I needed to ease the symptoms at any cost, no matter its causes.

That is how I started a pilgrimage along the route of non-conventional medicine.

I tried yoga, but I felt frustrated since I could not follow the postures, I was as flexible as a rusted robot without WB40, and ended up with a contracture that did not let me move my neck.

So I went to acupressure, and got asleep, but once I woke up, so did SOM.

Then I tried with the chiropractic which was wonderful, but after the massive manipulation of my joints, I was bent as an origami swan.

My visit to the Chiropractic, which perform a treatment of the musculoskeletal system, especially the spine, under the belief that these disorders affect general health via the nervous system, was quite disturbing.

What really unnerved me, was the abrupt sound of cracking bones. It sounded like an endless chain of "pop!" like the sound of a machine gun.

When the Chiropractic ran out of ammo, and the session ended, I asked: "What was that sound? Don't worry -he said. When a joint is opened up, gas is released. Gas? –I said- and I came here thinking that the problem was my eye!"

It was time to give homeopathy a chance.

When I told the Homeopath about SOM, I could notice a combination gesture of surprise, curiosity and puzzlement.

He brought a book, which looked like a wizard's spelling book, a heavy and old ancient spirit book. I even was expecting him to blow the dust off the leather cover.

He uses his fingers to follow the –I guess- a list of different pathologies, trying to find mine.

After looking the old book, he said, "Trembling eyelid? Nope -I said." And he replied "Well it is close enough, let's try this". He looked at the book again, and prescribed some pills.

I bought those pills, and in order to make it as unnoticeable as possible, I put the homeopathic pills in an empty pack of tic-tacs.

This idea –for which I can only be compared to the genius of Da Vinci- would, in theory, let me discreetly take the pills at work.

Well, it did not work.

Unfortunately the pills were so tiny that the first time I tried it, my eye was shaking, and I spilled them all over the floor.

It was pathetic, I can tell you that. I found myself running after the rolling pills that were heading right to the printer in the middle of the office.

It was a sad day in the evolutionary spiral of the humanity…

Finally, I went to acupuncture.

It was my first time, and I did not know what to expect, except of being greeted by a friendly aged Chinese person.

But when the curtain drew open, a man came slowly and he happened to totally look like Mao Tse-tung!

I immediately, tried to conceal any signal of shock that my face could express, while making an effort not to run away.

The man had a very severe look and seldom say a word, just "what's the problem" and "lay down on the stretcher".

He started needling. He started nice and easy, I should say. But after a few minutes, I began to feel some discomfort.

"I guess, that should be enough –I thought."

But no, he seemed resolute and absolutely committed to inflict as much pain as possible. He went on, and on and on... like an inquisition's sadomasochistic fanatic.

I ended up like Pinhead (the sordid character of the Clive Barker's movie "Hellraiser") full of needles all over my face.

"Are you OK? –he asked. No! -I yell- Are you doing your needles thing, or are you throwing darts at me?!"

I wonder who said that acupuncture is not painful?

It seems that this practice was founded on statistical probability: the more needles one could stand, the higher the probability that at least one could get on the right spot.

I did not want more piercing, and I said goodbye for good, claiming irreconcilable differences.

In retrospect, it was a very interesting experience. After all, not everybody have the chance to meet "Vlad the Impaler".

At that point, I needed both: to mitigate SOM and to fix everything broken, bent, and punched all along my previous tryouts.

I needed a break and a quote of self-indulgence. So my next step, was trying the physiotherapist, and you know? It worked.

I got so relaxed that I could put my mind at ease; and once the session ended, SOM symptoms were gone, for the first time in a long, long time.

Since then I love having a good massage, and I keep having two massage sessions a month for therapeutic purposes.

It is quite pricey, but hey! It make no sense taking more care for your car to extend its life, than you do for extend yours.

I really do not know… Perhaps it is not that these therapies were worthless, but I was not ready and receptive to take advantage of them. Or perhaps I simply did not go to the best specialists.

At any rate, I had to keep on with my epic fight against SOM, once again and by my own.

It was kind of ironic… I work on quality management, but I was not able to provide me with some quality of life.

CHAPTER 3.
AT WORK

As a Quality Management professional, my performance is closely tied to my eyesight, as quality depends on the attention to details, and details rely on paying attention.

Perhaps it could not be fair to say that my job is especially susceptible to SOM, when there are jobs even more dependent on view sight, such as drivers, pilots or surgeons. I used to think that being SOM such a problem to me, it must be impossible for them.

No matter how dependable your job is, SOM is debilitating and restrictive.

I realized that my own condition started at work, was triggered there and at some extent ended there too.

GETTING OUT FROM THE FUNHOUSE TUNNEL

Commuting

What an dramatic irony getting a Kindle to avoid carrying lots of books (I like to read many simultaneously) and not being able to use it anymore.

One day, going to work, an episode of The Twilight Zone came to my mind. It was an episode filmed in 1959, that freaked me out when I was about 10 years old. It was something like this:

Bank teller and avid bookworm, Henry Bemis takes his lunch break in the bank's vault, where his reading will not be disturbed.

Moments after he sees a newspaper headline, which reads "H-Bomb Capable of destruction", an explosion outside the bank shakes the vault, knocking Bemis unconscious.

After regaining consciousness and recovering the thick glasses he needed, Bemis emerges from the vault, to find the bank demolished and everyone in it dead.

Leaving the bank, he sees that the entire city has also been destroyed and realizes that a nuclear war has devastated the Earth but that his being in the vault has saved him.

Absolutely alone in a shattered world with food to last him a lifetime, but no one to share it with, Bemis succumbs to despair.

As he prepares to commit suicide using a revolver he has found, Bemis sees the ruins of the public library in the distance.

He finds that all the books he could ever hope for are his for reading, and all the time in the world to read them without interruption.

His despair gone, Bemis contentedly sorts the books he looks forward to reading, for years to come.

Just as he bends down to pick up the first book, he stumbles, and his glasses fall off and shatter.

In shock, he picks up the broken remains of the glasses he is virtually blind without, and says, "That is not fair. That is not fair at all!", and bursts into tears, surrounded by books he now can never read.

It was not until a few years ago that after recalling this episode in the midst of a terrible SOMday, I found it on Internet and learned it was one of the most famous episodes of the whole show. Even Rod Serling –the author of the episode and creator of the show- cited the episode as being one of his two favorites from the entire series.

As an avid reader, I felt myself as Mr. Bemis.

I used to take advantage the long commuting way in the subway to read. Two hours just for me, my own vault of 20.5 kilometers long where I could dedicate myself to reading. It may seem not that much, but it is about 30 days of continuous reading in a year.

Since I was sharing the place with other 345 thousand travelers, it was not my space for sure, not even a pleasant one in those crowded 40 years-old cars without an air conditioner, but, it was my time, with no role other than being a reader.

GETTING OUT FROM THE FUNHOUSE TUNNEL

There, I was not to play the role of a father, nor a husband, nor a son or a neighbor. I was not the well-known professional or the employee I had to be for at least the following 10 hours.

But SOM ripped it out from me as I found impossible to keep reading because of the movement of the train, the jerk of my eye and the dizziness.

The subway with the fluorescent lights became a tricky extension of the funhouse tunnel.

During a reading, every time I finished a sentence, I got lost and lose the next line to maintain a flowing smooth reading.

In Buenos Aires, getting to work is already a stressful and unhealthy experience.

To the natural uncertainty of living in Argentina, you have to add that your day begins not knowing if the already mediocre transportation system would work because of technical issues, chronic union strikes or any other excuse.

You start the day wondering if the daily barricades or the multiple popular manifestations, pro or against any cause, would let you go through, all of this sick context would affect even more the drivers and walkers until the point of boiling.

You do not know if it would be prudent to expose yourself to the smugglers and marginal people that almost took over the city.

At some point, you will question the commutefulness: whether it is worth commuting to the office and you will question whether all those face time or those days with little work to do or a lot of it but with no need of personal interaction worth the distress of the trip.

Living in the XXI century is so easy to telecommuting or teleworking from home; I barely understand the old school boys that need to see their army of employees to their own rejoice and self-admiration.

In a world when information can travel at light speed across the globe, why do people have to travel every single day even if that is not necessary at all if it is about processing and developing information?

In times of crisis, how much would be saved if companies would not have to build massive facilities.

How much money could be save from providing a corporate space to every single employee, paying for it, its maintenance and assurance as it would be used 24 hours a day and the 365 days of the year (including night hours, weekends, holidays and other conventional non-productive time).

Hoteling is a form of providing unassigned seating in an office. It like hot desking, but hoteling is reservation-based unassigned seating, whereas, hot desking is reservation-less unassigned work places.

I advocate these methods based on economical, ecological, contingency and human rationales.

A few years ago, I initiated the teleworking initiative. It grew to corporate levels and led to a governmental agreement to promote it.

Unfortunately, this kind of initiatives used to be seen as trivial and worthless, and of course they are if it is not deployed with a critical mass of employees which resulted in room and costs savings.

Some managers claim that teleworking are not for everyone and suspect an underperformance of their teams. Truth is that teleworking is not for every employee or job, but in my experience those who need a deeper mental shift are the management itself.

Even if teleworking is not a philosophy that your company formally adheres, sometimes it is up to your boss and his willing to increase his freedom of choice, in situations where previously he thought he had little or none.

That is, of course, based on the premise that you have the discipline to organize your working day at home in order to get a work-life balance and maintain a healthy relationship with your boss.

Relationships

Ultimately –after all the tribulations of commuting- you get your way to your work, already tired and stressed, and the big shots using the company cars obviously do not understand you.

As you cannot imagine that other colleagues have a longer trip than you, as a long string of broken links of disconnected people that ignores and do not give a damn to other sacrifices or miseries are built.

But not everybody is like that, maybe you are different, and care for your colleagues and the members of your teamwork.

Perhaps you fight against the unstoppable forces of sociopaths that channel all their personal and professional frustration, bawling and snapping at an innocent person or creature who just happens to be handy.

Following a lousy day at work, even if you cannot take it out on your boss; perhaps you are one of those strange birds that make the rational decision in order to avoid kicking the cat.

The problem is that even you were proud of your ethical position; chances are that you would be de center of a vortex of stress, so you have to find a way to release the pressures that you accumulate and absorb in the sake of others and mainly in order to live on your own standards.

Eventually I was forced to soak up and work under so much emotional pressure that at the end of the day I felt my trip back to home, as a virtual deck decompression chamber.

You may know it for sure, or you may suppose it, but in a corporate environment people are known for their profile as hunters or shepherds.

It seems that SOM tends to affect those shepherds that pretend to be a hunter in the sake of their careers.

Recognizing yourself as a shepherd or hunter is essential, because being consistent with yourself is imperative to stress release.

Whether it is because fear, vanity or survival, you may think that the best thing to do is to pretend that everything is just fine, masking your SOM, hiding its symptoms at all costs.

You may think you should to hide your situation to your boss, perhaps you also think it would be convenient to do it with your pals too.

In my experience continuously hiding my SOM to everyone, resulted to be exhausting and almost futile. And it seems pretty counterfeit.

If others do not know what it is, they will believe what is not. Some ticks you may get because of SOM effects may be seen quite weird. It is hard enough dealing with SOM as force yourself pretending a lie in your working life.

Of course, it is not a matter of hung a banner saying how proud or sad you are, but to release some tension looking for a good confident, a trusted person to share your real experience.

No matter what my job is, I always respect everyone and enjoy conversations with security guards, assistants, janitors, drivers and anyone whom may show something interesting to talk about. It keeps me rooted and centered, being aware of other people realities.

Sincere care or attention to others happens to be reciprocal. If you are glad to other people's achievement or sincerely sorry for their problems, most probably you will find that the other is willing to listen to you too.

I discovered it, while in the midst of a bad moment in life.

Once a month, I order from home two ice-creams for my wife and me. I was unemployed and we granted the privilege of give ourselves some self-indulgence. I used to choose not to buy a bigger ice cream, in order to afford a third one for Charlie, the doorman.

He was a very likeable person, a veteran of war forced to fight when he was just a teenager.

One night, after a lousy day looking for a job, I returned home very sad and tired. It was not our ice-cream night, but there he was Charlie at the door with ice-cream for us.

Perhaps you may think that you do not have right to whining to less fortunate people in the "social ladder". But that is a convention and an illusion that makes us believe that the higher you are the happier you will become.

There is no rule for that, but as I have been at the bottom and later rose above, I am aware that from the bottom sometimes you can judge the terms of the tradeoff of being at the top as quite destructive and unappealing.

Is there a person you can trust to share the basics of your experience with your eye? It really helps.

Just sharing what I was going through with a single person, helped me release a lot of pressure. In my case, it was the waiter that served the Directors.

Being at work counting with someone that truly ask you "how is your eye today?" is one of the most useful and valuable help I ever found at work.

Technology

One of the most basic nuisances I found was writing e-mail.

As the rush of the day requires prompt responses to answer all your mail, no matter how good reflex do you have to do it, or if you used to reply with tennis volley shot returning to the sender the requested response in mid-air before the mail bounces in your mail inbox, ultimately the jumping eye conspires against you.

SOM forces to double check everything, I could not trust on my own writing. No matter how many times I checked it, and how well the word process spell checker was, I always find a typo.

Moreover, spell checking is excellent, but takes time and at the very beginning I did not want to recognize I needed it (not because of the grammar but because of SOM).

With time, I learned to check my messages in other ways. I read the messages I sent during my first years of SOM, and they always have at least one instance of letter reversal.

It was like having dyslexia, and even though there is no cure for it, dyslexic individuals can learn to read and write with educational support through techniques that allow managing or evening concealing its symptoms.

And just as I found that like dyslexia, removing stress and anxiety alone can improve SOM effects.

Accepting and changing your compulsive e-mail immediate response habits, your real-time spell check would release some stress (not to mention it could improve the quality of the content of the message).

And for the Graham Bell's contentment, I started to use the phone again, which eventually was instrumental to improve relationships with co-workers.

Anyway, it was usual that, no matter how many times I checked a message, once sent I still found errors. Sometimes I could recover it, but sometimes I could not, then I hated the irony of being in a work context that was at least instrumental to cause SOM, and at the same time, preventing me to perform as I used to, as I wanted to, and as they demanded.

I have to design processes represented on complex drawings with thousands of vectors. A wrong arrow would indicate a wrong work routine, many of them with directions about processes in hazardous environments.

With time, I learned how to handle it with usual performance, even though I had to double check everything at home, or do whatever was necessary.

I can imagine what you could feel if your job involves driving, operating machinery, manipulation of hazardous chemicals, or requires a lot of precision.

By the way, when SOM shows, there was a tiny yet upsetting challenge: passwords!

OK, remembering all passwords is already difficult and could be frustrating enough, and it fiercely goes to another level when a password must meet higher complexity and length.

Long string of numbers, mix cases and symbols, makes a security measure into a torture and punishment.

One of the most annoying situation for me used to be login-in to the password protected printer at work through that the wicked virtual keyboard on the tiny touch screen.

Under normal circumstances, typing on the small virtual keys already required to use pen covers or – paradoxically- the corner of the company security pass card.

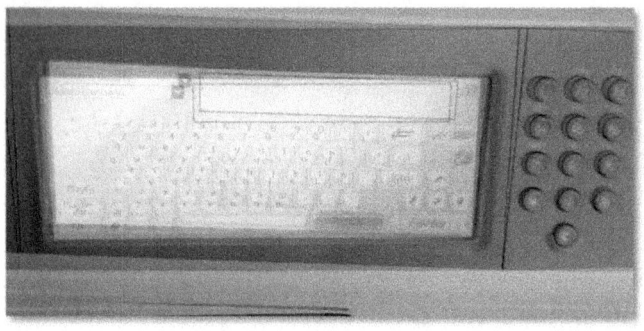

Picture 4: The challenging printer.

When everything is shaking, not even William Tell –the embodiment of precision and accuracy- would find more difficult to log-in than shooting with his crossbow the apple over his son's head.

The second bothersome situation was entering the Blackberry password.

Even though the physical keyboard seemed to be fairly accessible or SOM-friendly, it still was too small.

In addition, as a company gadget and in order to comply with information security standards, a time-out was set which forces the user to log-in after a certain time, which was a frequent nuisance (to say the least).

By the way, my SOM worsen as soon as my employer gave me a Blackberry.

An article in the British "The Telegraph", explored studies that revealed many employees were turning into workaholics because of the ability to receive and send messages and work online even when they were at home.

That staff with mobile technology such as Blackberries work an extra 15 hours a week as they constantly check emails even out of the office, according to new research.

Some agree, other do not. Some say that there is a 'downtime' during the day we can now make it more productive using that time to process e-mail. Some say that faffing with e-mail is not working, but just labor-saving technology making life harder. That is fine.

My viewpoint is quite easy to understand: there is nothing intrinsically good or bad, said that I have two questions:

Who benefits with your productivity during your 'downtime'. Do you think that a company would give a device to its employees because altruistic reasons?

No way. There have to be a return of the investment and it is quite naïve thinking otherwise.

But the fact is not whether you should use a smartphone or not but that you have to be aware if you are crossing that thin line between working and playing with a new gadget.

Be conscious of the new concept of "gamification" which is the use of game dynamics in a non-game context.

Do not get me wrong, I love technology and gadgets, but make sure high-tech is at your service and not the other way around, and work is not masked under the appearance of a game.

You have to take care of your eyes' health, either working or playing. Just be alert to physical signs that may warn you that reading and replying a bunch of messages in a tiny 2.64 inches display may cost an arm, a leg and an eye.

Making more productive your 'downtime' forcing your eyes while commuting, would demand to trade off your performance dealing with real people at your work place.

Meetings

Meetings use to start with introductions. No big deal, right? Well, if you have SOM, it certainly is.

Sometimes the anxiety got so severe, that I just wanted to be alone, and since that was not possible, I sat in meetings just wondering how the room would look like on a fire drill.

Eye contact occurs when people look at each other's nonverbal communication as a meaningful and important sign of confidence and social communication.

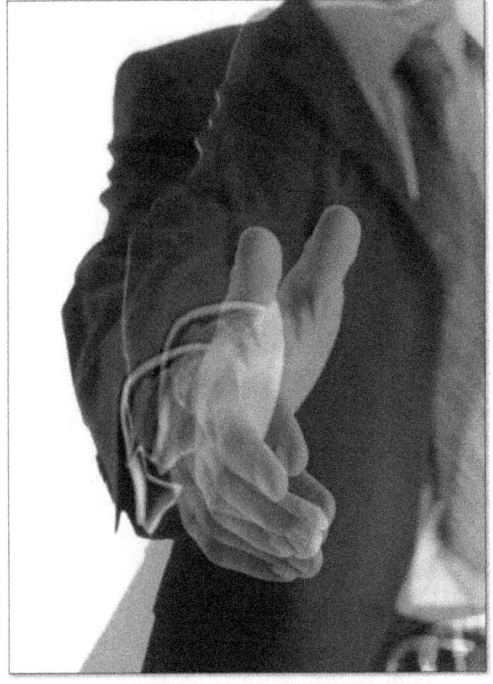

Picture 5: SOM puts the "shake" at the end of "handshake".

The constant shaking of your sight induces and at the same time affects you to make an effective eye contact. I found this extremely weaken and disturbing.

How come that even during a good SOMday, a casual meeting triggers the eye jerking?

Well, in a British study psychologists concluded that while humans obtain useful information from looking at the face when listening to someone, the process of looking at faces is mentally challenging and takes processing. Therefore, it even may be unhelpful to look at faces when trying to concentrate and process something else that is mentally demanding.

At the beginning, I thought that the trigger was the effort trying to sustain eye contact with a person standing too close, but it happens that eye contact may be stressing, and that was the actual hidden cause.

Since I was a teenager, I programmed myself to make eye contact with others. You know, all of us have its strengths and weaknesses to establish relations (and flirting). I realized that I had to take advantage of my communication skills becoming a champion of non-verbal communication.

But since SOM began I had to learn to relax. If this annoying condition is useful to something, it is to being aware of those things that push you beyond natural limits; even you consciously do not know it or accept it.

Now you know something they do not: looking right at the eyes of others, requires an unimagined effort, that if you can manage it, it will become an advantage to you.

As I learned how to make eye contact in the past, I learned how to do it calm and easy, on an undemanding way.

Until then, I manage to adopt a position that, in the most natural way as possible, let me occlude my bumping eye to ease the symptoms.

But that is not all.

The problem with SOM goes beyond the rotation of the eye. When it stops, it may do it on the original position or slightly twisted, which resulted on double vision.

So, during the shaking, I did not only beg it to stop, but to stop on its natural angle. If it did not, I was forced to quickly learn which image was the real one.

When I failed to so, I ended up seeing above their heads, instead of at their faces, and if that happened, they started to discreetly touch their hair, and eventually asking if they had something wrong there.

It used to be a real embarrassing moment for both.

Presentations

You were introduced; you are at some point in the meeting when you should present a slideshow.

Well, that can be a real threat to your career and reputation. No matter how well prepared you may be, it has an unquestionably share of stress and adrenaline.

Your heart starts pumping blood faster, your hands sweat, your mouth is dry, and the PowerPoint is ready to be shown. That is under normal conditions.

With SOM, you should add the fact that the entire meeting room is shaking, and if not yet, you should be ready to be near San Andreas Fault.

Let put it this way:

You are presenting your slideshow.

Suddenly, the whole room twists clockwise about 30 degrees. The entire audience, the meeting table and everything in front of you seem to be launched from a slingshot like angry birds.

I noticed that the more time SOM took to show itself, the further the imaginary slingshot was pulled back, resulting in a more fierce effect.

Then the whole room violently returns back, but during the spin, you do not only are confused by the motion, but by a double image that comes and goes.

Your eye twist back and forth, repeating this phenomenon like a perpetual motion machine.

You try to keep calm, but the more you try, the hardier it becomes to control it.

You start to feel dizzy and disoriented, but you stand still, stoical and indomitable, (perhaps cursing your eye) but still pretending everything is OK.

Before SOM, I did not realize that presentations were shown at smaller surfaces.

With projectors, there was more space than with a TV, which is the actual standard.

I used to love that change, but with SOM it poses a new challenge: even though presentations now could be more visually appealing, the font sizes are quite difficult to read if you are on the opposite side of the meeting table.

I never like to read presentations, preferring visual triggers or keywords to long texts, but even the most concise slideshow may require hyperlinks, and that is when problems arise.

I knew my speech, I had the information, the presentation was impressive, but when I had to click on the link, to go to another slide, I could not do it because the whole thing was shaking like crazy.

I had to improvise saying something like "look closely at the figure on the second row!"; so when the audience turned their heads towards the screen, I could close my eye (as winking) and then, without the shakiness and double vision, I could drag the cursor right over the link and click on it.

Since then, I changed the way I design my presentations, avoiding anything that may need precision, making sequential and continuous slides replacing regular hyperlinks on words or small buttons with large transparent areas.

One time, I was so drained because SOM, that I made the executive presentation to the board of director with a brand new design. Instead of overloaded spreadsheets, I designed what I announced as a minimalist presentation. Each slide looked as an Apple add. They liked it. I would have never dared to do it before SOM.

Business trips

Either in the sake of the company resources as for a work/home balance, I have never been loose on flying when it is not required.

Some time ago, a boss urged me that I should fly somewhere, without any particular reason but to being seen.

I said that I rather stay.

He asked me "Is that are you afraid of airplanes?" To which I replied "I am not afraid of airplanes, but just of the idea of free falling".

Once in a while I had to take a flight, and when justified, I am always willing.

However, since SOM began, the trembling eye, plus turbulence and the usual lightheadedness made me feel like if all the plane were spinning. Really awful indeed.

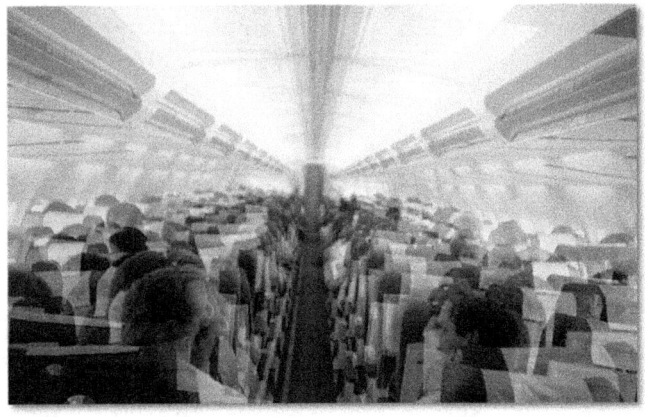

Picture 6: Airplane! With SOM it is a matter of both fight and fly!

Business as usual

I remember SOMdays so tough that, I hardly could pretend that everything was OK.

As soon as I had a chance, I ran through a seeming rotating and shaking corridor, feeling my way along the walls to get to the restroom. Then I got into the bathroom stall and locked the door sobbing and begging it stops. That is the humiliating truth about why I went out from the office so often.

Sometimes I wanted it to stop it so badly I wished my eyeball to be lifted out of its socket. Of course, this thought did not last for more than a few microseconds; but I still had it.

A SOMday reminded me the viral video "Harlem Shake". It usually began quite calm, with one person dancing to the song alone, surrounded by other people not paying attention or seemingly unaware of the dancing individual, and when the bass drops, the video cuts to the entire crowd, doing a crazy convulsive dance.

Same as my eye, it could be relatively nice, with little or none tremors at all, and unexpectedly exploding into an uncontrolled shaking, making everything seems to jump around me.

I used to say "when the problem is in your eye, the pain is in your neck" (and I mean it, literally).

To soften SOM symptoms and keep working with the computer, without even notice it, I found a position in which my eye did not go wild. So I found myself instinctively adopting a crooked position.

It was something like this:

I slightly tilted my head to the left (getting the left ear closer to the left shoulder), then I faintly moved my head downwards (bringing my chin to my chest) and I kept my eyes looking a little bit upper the horizon (as looking your "third eye" during a meditation).

The result? I ended up looking as Jack Nicholson, lifting his eyebrows totally crazy in The Shining movie.

Unfortunately, this posture was not SOM-proof, and the eye eventually used to move and stop at a weird position. To "unlock" it, I had to blink and unconsciously join the blinking with a movement of my head to the left, which looked as tics and twitches.

This ludicrous position and movement, plus sitting on a chair in the wrong position (with my back bent towards the desk, instead of being straight) resulted on a real pain the neck (I am not kidding!).

I had muscle spasms, backache, cricks in my neck, headache and dizziness –usually when I stand up after a long period of staring at the monitor. I barely could last out, until the end of the work day.

That abrupt vertigo terrified me so much that ignited a scary slippery slope; with a quick lowering of the blood pressure, feeling that I was going to lose consciousness and a strange feeling of being detached from myself, and then I got scared to death, which caused me a sudden rise of blood pressure and an abnormally rapid heartbeat:

I did not know yet, but was already applying to the Panic Attack Club.

Mitigating the problem

My SOM began at work. It surely had several triggers, but incidentally, as most of the people that intensively use computer and other digital devices; I experienced symptoms of Computer Vision Syndrome (CVS).

These are the actions I took to ease it:

1.   Got a thorough eye exam.

First I needed to dismiss any problem, checking my eyes with a professional. I asked him if my eyeglasses could be customized for computer use.

I tried wearing anti-reflective (AR) glasses, but it did not help that much.

2. Set the lighting, avoiding glare:

The bright light from outdoor sunlight coming in through a window was just terrible. No matter how "smart" the building may be, the window walls make the room too bright, not to mention when the sun gets reflected on the river.

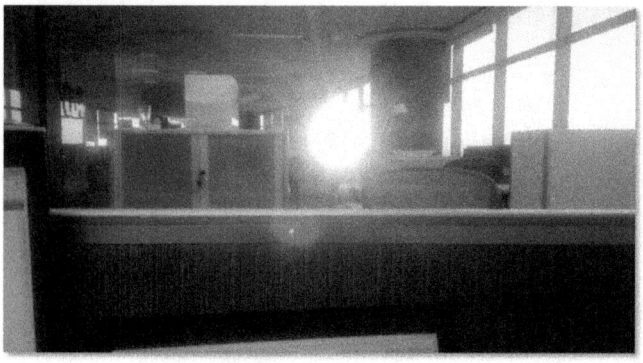

Picture 7: Beautiful sunrise at the office... except for the glare.

Shades were too translucent and insufficient to block the outside light.

I tried to avoid placing my PC screen in front or behind it.

Since there was no independent switch to turn them off, I requested to take the overhead fluorescent tubes trying to reduce the overhead lighting.

I moved to a darker spot of the office.

As if it would not have been enough, window walls of the management offices were right in front of the outer window walls, reflecting the light on my screen.

And to embellish the concrete walls, yellow tinted glass panels were installed here and there.

3. Upgraded the display and adjusted the settings.

The new wide-screen monitors with a flat-panel liquid crystal display (LCD) were a pleasant surprise when we moved to the new building.

It was a large display, and I set it to the maximum resolution and the font size a little but larger to reduce the effort and fatigue.

I adjusted the text size and contrast for comfort, especially because I like to write with a two pages view of the document. Black font on a white background is the combination I always choose.

I tried to adjust the brightness if it looks like a white paper.

4. ExercEyes

I relaxed my eyes' muscles by shutting them tightly and relaxing them for a little time.

I changed my focus often, looking in another direction, getting up and choosing a relaxing landscape (where available), stretching the range of vision as far as possible to the right, to the left, down and up.

Blinking could stop the rotation movement of the eye.

I wondered if it related with eye strain and dry eyes. It made sense since the situation worsens with heat air conditioner, poor ventilated rooms, and steering long times at the monitor screen.

I forced myself to blink since I noticed that I did it not so often. So I started to do it on purpose.

My eye doctor prescribed artificial tears for use during the day. It was not a any regular product, but a special one which was more oily and dense. It really reduced dryness and irritation. At night, I used another one, which, in fact, is a gel.

Computer eyestrain caused focusing fatigue, forcing the eyes by constantly focusing on your screen. I forced myself to look away from your computer every now and then, and look a relaxed view such a park.

This exercises reduces the risk of focusing ability to "lock up" or accommodative spasm, after a long computer work.

I used to take breaks, you can use software to remind you to do so.

The neck, back and shoulder pain were quite strong and permanent because of the weird posture I set to minimize SOM. Shoulder blades pain was awful. I felt as the hunchback of Notre Dame.

Finally, I had to pay attention to correct my posture, being aware of incorrect position, correcting it whenever was necessary.

You may think that your eyes are firmly attached to muscles with chains. Let your eyeball free! Visualize it is floating freely as levitating. It helped me to learn how to relax every muscle of your face and your eyes.

If the eye moved, it was ok, if it was not, it was ok too. The goal was to be as relaxed as possible.

Relax your forehead, eyebrows, raising them gently and then letting them go back slowly.

Smile, the muscles of your cheeks will massage those of your eyes and bottom eyelids and is proven that even a fake smile triggers the same hormones as an honest one.

"Take that look from your face." Do it in a Tai-chi pace. At bullet speed.

If you cannot swim, sit on the floor with your legs crossed and move your arms as if swimming and back style. Watch your style; you will become the dry Stephen Phelps. Rotate your joints. Stretch your arms until your fingertips. Feel your shoulder blades moves as the muscles of your neck stretches out.

5. Go outdoors.

Frequent breaks during the work day were necessary, at least short breaks to stand up, go around and stretch every limb, neck, back and shoulders.

There is a world out there. I learned that if I spend my lunch time outdoors, instead of still working, the world will keep going around and the building will not tilt 15 degrees to the right.

Enjoy the natural light a few times during the day. I used to go out from the office and walk around a nearby park.

Fresh air relaxing and taking some stress out from my mind. Look at the top of the trees, and breathe.

* * *

You can find more information about How to stop eye twitching at **http://www.wikihow.com/Stop-Eye-Twitching**

CHAPTER 4.
AT HOME

"It is easy to fool the eye, but it is hard to fool the heart." Al Pacino

* * *

Your home should be your castle, your palace, your temple and your shelter.

After a bad SOMday, I could not wait to get home and relax, release some strain from my eyes with drops, water and a cold gel mask with which I resemble a retired superhero.

But, as SOM worsen, and dizziness and vertigo used to take over my work day, I began experiencing collateral effects which affected me even at home: I was secretly afraid.

First, I was afraid to do some task, like doing home improvement with the driller or other precision tools.

Later, after a violent movement of my eye during a shower, when I lost some balance, I was even afraid of fainting on the bath.

Finally, I was so fearful; I was unsure of my own capacity to take care of my kids. I needed my wife to stay with me just in case something happen to me.

I started avoiding outdoor activities, such riding bikes or fly kites. Later, I did not even go to the movies.

It was not just the possibility of enjoy because of the symptoms, but a real worry about "what would happen to my kids if something bad occurs to me?".

As a XXI century dad, I have always pleased of join my kids everywhere and being a present father, attentive to their school, attending to their concerts, bringing them to the doctor, birthdays, and so on.

But SOM beat me hard on this, and I just avoided being alone with them, losing all the joy that it meant to me, crumbling my self-esteem as I felt myself unable to take care of them.

I could not even enjoy my kids as I used to do.

I have never missed their first-school day, and the first year with SOM, it was so aggressive that I was mad and the uncertainty of the condition terrified me.

I felt vulnerable, ashamed, frustrated and discombobulated.

The more I tried to resist it, the more focused I was on my SOM, instead of the moment I was supposed to be enjoying.

Until I got SOM, as soon as I got home, I used to play with my kids, dinner, tell my kids stories, take a shower, turn on my PC and work and study until late at night. Once I got SOM, not anymore.

My daughter loves singing and acting, and I am quite emotional especially when I see her doing her "shows".

The first year of my SOM experience, I went to her school concert, but, because of SOM, I could not even recognize her.

At that time I got deeply embittered and resentful.

Holidays

Holidays and parties lost their joy, even SOM may let me alone for a moment, internally I was still tense, and eventually it brutally appeared, preventing me to celebrate anything.

I recall doing my best trying to focus on the moment, but the constant shakiness of the eyes always drove me to curse SOM and all its triggers for the precious moments I was missing.

No matter the celebration, I got to a point when I screwed my face into a grimace of disgust.

It is interesting, though, how you take things for granted until you lose it, and in relation to SOM, is a revelation being aware how we take our vision and balance for granted.

How could my friends understand that I was happy to join their Xmas dinner, although my expression was as if I was disgusting or annoyed?

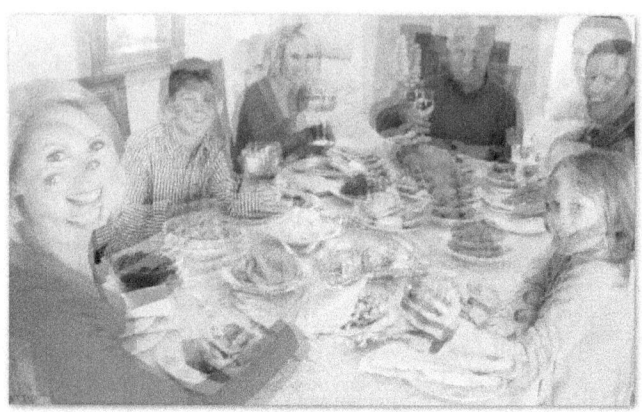

Picture 8: Not so merry Xmas...

How could ever my family understand that it was my eye that was spinning, not the dreidel?! (dreidel is the four-sided spinning top, played with during the Jewish holiday of Hanukkah).

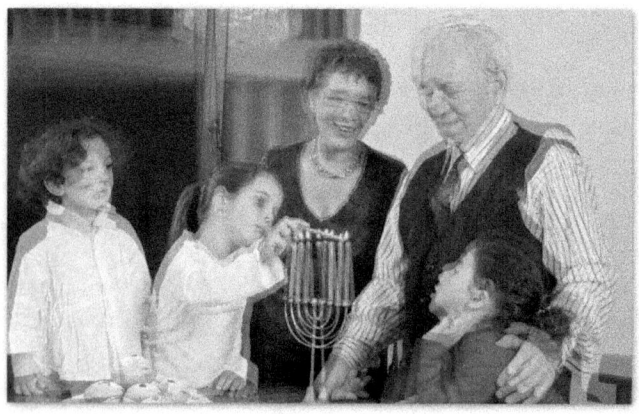

Picture 9: SOM turned off the Festival of Lights

How to avoid wishing that the next year SOM – somehow- stops, once and for all?

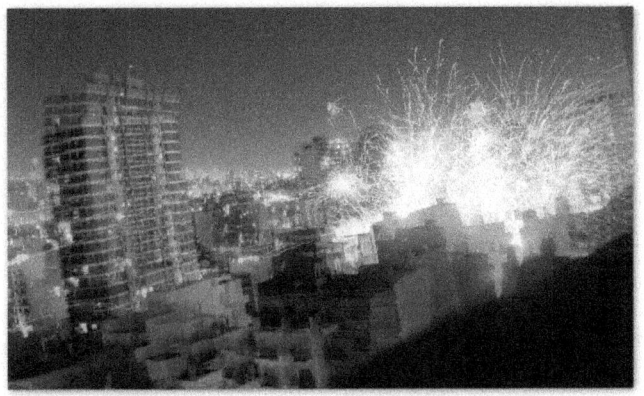

Picture 10: New Year's Eve in Buenos Aires

TV (not that it worth that much, though)

Since SOM, I kept me away from any screen. I stopped watching TV, working and studying got extremely difficult both with digital and printed material and I absolutely avoided my PC, which was always a tool as well as and entertainment in those moments when the family was sleeping, and I was with some privacy and quietness.

With SOM, even if I got the time, it was worthless. Trying to focus on the TV screen triggered my eye shaking.

Shockingly, everything worsen when I watched the news. I recalled that my eye got exceedingly violent during the broadcast of the 2011 earthquake off the Pacific coast of Tōhoku. When I watched a father crying for his son, over the ruins of a day care house swept by the tsunami, I felt I was there (I genuinely felt his sorrow), and everything frantically twitched all around me.

The wild behavior of my eye continued later on, during the Fukushima tension to shut down the nuclear plant.

The correlation between my mood and SOM became quite evident.

Enjoying a DVD used to be difficult enough with two demanding kids. I barely had time to watch anything except children movies.

Watching movies required effort, the only positive thing was that I had no choice but listening the original audio (instead of reading the subtitles), which helped me practice my English.

But one of the most disturbing things that ever happened during my SOM journey, was the finding of the personal diary of my great-great-grandfather.

I found it (my hobby used to be genealogy) and as read its pages, I stopped in the year 1883.

This is what he wrote: "Then, my mother was not at home but in Konigsberg with my little sister Miriam that needed an eye surgery. They stayed there a few months, it was cancer. She got her eye removed and replaced it with a glass eye."

"What the heck?! –I though."

If this is sad for any sensitive person, if that person is a relative it becomes gloomier, if this relative is also hypochondriac it becomes a warning notice, and if that hypochondriac, is also a SOMer this story becomes whether consciously or not, a terrifying probability.

Hobbies

I have a small balcony, with more than 60 plants. I like gardening and with SOM it was difficult to enjoy it.

I sat out there and tried to feel de warm sunshine on my face, smelling the flowers, hearing the birds, feeling the breeze and touching the soil which helped me out to get some peace at harsh moments and eventually SOM symptoms started to drop.

I realized that most of my joy depended on the visual sense. I strove to learn how to widen the scope of enjoyment to new senses.

That is why I also learned to play guitar. I always wanted to play a musical instrument, and guitar happened to be wonderful.

I found that not only the sound of the most basic arpeggios was totally relaxing, but also de vibration of the instrument over the chest helped to induce a state of relaxation and in addition learning something new, fed my self-respect proving to be able to perform new faculties.

I also love drawing. At the begging, while fighting against SOM, I got tense and could not draw a single sketch.

Later, I kept alone late at night, with soft music, trying to surrender to SOM and let it flow. Then as someone that is urged to say something brief and then chooses for silence, SOM vanished with each single trace of the pencil. I let it come. I let it go.

Sports

I was eager to swim, and I dared to jump into the swimming pool. I was afraid something happened during the swimming, but I found that the exercise on water helped me to get a high level of comfort.

I loved it so much it made me feel so good, I –as never before- swam every single day.

After a few weeks, it seemed that the goggles I wore stopped SOM symptoms. Once I putted them on, the shakiness stopped, but I am not quite sure whether it was because the pressure of the goggles on my eyes muscles or an emotional anchor that attached the relaxation feeling with the fact of wearing them.

I did not dare, though, to make an underwater turn because I was afraid of losing the sense of orientation.

I swam daily, nice and easy, just breaststroke to limited the eye movements, and on those times where the swimming pool was almost empty (the echoes of the constant noises when the pool were full of people did not let me relax as much as I needed).

Swimming was fantastic: I got some time off from the SOM symptoms; I release endorphins which made me feel great, and it was like a massage that helped to the back and neck ache I had because the strange positions I have been adopting to counterbalance the grim vision.

No matter how tired or lazy I was, I went swimming and sometime later, even the smell of the Clorox, eased my SOM.

At some point, I was feeling so good I tried the bike again and guess what? It was quite OK. So I kept biking and swimming, and for the first time in my life I participated on a city alley cat race.

Food

At the beginning I felt so intoxicated because a bad diet, I needed a sweeping change.

I engaged into a detox diet with just fruits and veggies juice, later fruits and veggies in solid state, and finally adding some fish, nuts, rice and other foods.

I thought that this was going to be healthy, plus, avoiding any hidden transgenic food, would prevent SOM in case it is triggered by an allergy.

So I gave the Soylent Green a break and started a healthy diet. I lost about 45 pounds! And I felt better than ever!

Protecting the eyes starts with the food on the plate. Studies have shown that nutrients such as omega-3 fatty acids, lutein, zinc, and vitamins C and E may help ward off age-related vision problems.

Research shows that eyes need vitamins, especially antioxidant vitamins A, C and E to be included in everyday diet.

Among every vitamin, for SOM there could be a must to take: Vitamin E. Based on what I studied to relieve SOM, lack of it produces neurological problems in the eyes and the whole body due to poor nerve conduction.

Even tears which are made up of water, mucus, and fat, require high quality Omega 3, 6 and 9 oils and a lot of water, to facilitate your eyes moist.

I ate foods that lead to eye health, such: Green, leafy vegetables such as spinach and collards. Salmon, tuna, and other oily fish. Eggs, nuts, beans, and other non-meat protein sources. Oranges and other citrus fruits or juices.

I am not quite sure if the food had a direct influence reducing SOM symptoms, but I certainly looked and felt great!

These are the fruits, vegetables and grains I took, in view of their effects on eye health:

VITAMIN A

* Carrot

* Broccoli leaf

* Sweet potato

* Kale
* Spinach
* Pumpkin
* Collard greens
* Cantaloupe/Melon
* Spinach

LUTEIN

* Kale
* Spinach
* Peas
* Zucchini
* Brussels sprouts
* Pistachios
* Broccoli
* Corn

VITAMIN C

* Rose hip
* Gooseberry
* Blackcurrant
* Red pepper
* Parsley

* Guava
* Kiwi
* Broccoli
* Loganberry
* Redcurrant
* Brussels sprouts
* Lychee

VITAMIN E

* Wheat germ oil
* Almonds
* Sunflower seeds
* Sunflower oil
* Hazelnuts
* Peanuts
* Spinach
* Broccoli
* Soybean oil
* Kiwi
* Mango
* Tomato
* Spinach

Sleeping

"Every closed eye is not sleeping, and every open eye is not seeing." Bill Cosby

* * *

I recalled being troubled about sleeping because of two issues:

First: even shutting my eyes I could not reduce SOM. I even began dreaming of trembling situations, just as those awake. I used to have nightmares about it.

Second: I was afraid to wake up and open my eyes just to find a shakiness vision (because it happened several times, and it was an extremely disturbing way to start the day).

Sometimes, I woke up with eye fatigue as if I were moving my eyes all night while I was sleeping, which resulted in sleep deprivation. The normal stage of sleep with rapid eye movement (REM)? SOM? Both? I never knew.

As I brushed my teeth, I used to spend a lot of time looking at my eye on the mirror, trying to find what was wrong with it.

The fact is that my first thought in the morning, and last thought at night, was about my wild eye.

SOM became a big black hole, that used to swallowed any other aspect of my life.

Night guards

"No man knows till he has suffered from the night how sweet and dear to his heart and eye the morning can be." Bram Stoker

* * *

In the sake of release some tension, I investigated and found that there was a syndrome linked to high levels of stress, can cause headaches, vision and hearing problems, and tooth damage: TMJ (Temporo-Mandibular Joint).

Simply stated, this is your jaw joint; the area where your lower jaw (mandibular) attaches to the skull at the temporal bone.

We have two TMJ's – one on each side although they work together.

For TMJ treatment, mouth guards, including night guards and orthotics devices or "bite splints," are non-invasive plastic objects that happen to relieve pain, prevent damaging behaviors and gently fix the misaligned bite over time.

There are two types of mouthguards: Night guards and splints.

Night guards are dental appliances made of soft plastic that fit over some or all of the teeth and are worn only during sleep to prevent tooth grinding, protect the teeth from wear and tear and relax the jaw.

These night guards are available in a wide range of prices, from a very inexpensive model that can be purchased at any drugstore to a customized model designed to fit your teeth precisely.

Custom-fit night guards are more effective than cheap over-the-counter guards.

They are also more comfortable to wear, which in turn encourages more regular use.

You are so stiff that eventually your expression lines seems a rock as if you have applied an overdose of Botox, and your frowning seems to stay petrified.

Frozen gel mask

The eye mask is a plastic eye mask shaped to fit over the eyes with gel inside it, very useful to treat red or swollen eyes caused by extended eye strain.

Frequent use of a gel eye mask helped relieve some of the symptoms associated with strain or lack of sleep.

Cool gel eyes patch soothed tired eyes, reduce puffiness and relieve stress and moist compresses helped relieve the pain, but those were not enough.

Placing a cool eye mask over the eyes helped soothe my tired or strained eyes and reduced the pain around the eyes, behind the eyelids and fatigue after a hard SOMday.

I used it cold and overnight, allowing coolness of the mask to reach the eyelids and the surrounding skin.

It was really good (even though my daughter used to tell me that I looked as the cousin of Mr. Incredible).

Eye patch

I thought I had to give a try something more radical such an eye patch, so I wondered all through the city looking for it.

Nobody knew I tried that one.

I looked at myself with the eye patch in the mirror. I felt so strange! I did not know whether I was missing my eye, the hook or parrot.

Even the results were satisfactory, I did not feel confident enough as to wear it in public, not to mention revealing my little secret at work. So I throw it away.

Gratifications

One day, after countless visits to the neuro-ophthalmologist, I returned home without any solution or tip to relieve my SOM (again).

So, I got home, and my wife straightaway asked:

- What did the doctor say?

-Honey -I said- I know it may sound weird, but the doctor prescribed sexual intercourse.

Puzzled, she asked: -will it really help you out with your eye?

-Not really, but at least I am going to have a helluva night!

It does not matter, where or how you find joy, diversion, happiness or bliss, what I learned is that in order to release some pressure, you have to get some pleasure.

You will not get the exit, walking on hot coals, laying on a bed of nails or eating fire.

You are suffering enough already, and you are guilty of nothing as to expect that the way out of this situation is through mental or physical self-flagellation.

It was very hard, but later on I realized that was wrong.

I used to think that I would be happy once I get rid of SOM, but the truth was that SOM started to go away, when I learned to enjoy little things again.

Enjoy life in your way.

SIMON BEIDER

CHAPTER 5.
ON THE STREET

Driving

"I have only one eye. Do you want me to look at the road or at the speedometer?" Moshe Dayan

* * *

I could not express it better than it is in the website of the U.S. Department of Transportation National Highway Traffic Safety Administration (NHTSA):

"For most people, driving represents freedom, control and independence. Driving enables most people to get to the places they want or need to go. For many people, driving is important economically – some drive as part of their job or to get to and from work.

Driving is a complex skill. Our ability to drive safely can be affected by changes in our physical, emotional and mental condition."

You can keep your independence even if you have to cut back or give up on your driving. It may take planning ahead, but it will get you there.

Take in mind, rides with family and friends; taxi cabs; shuttle buses or vans; public buses, trains and subways.

Also, senior centers and religious and other local service groups often offer transportation services for older adults in the community.

The possibility of being unable to drive and loose that freedom of movement was awful. I just finished paying the last payment of my car when SOM began.

I had my first car at age 33, and I felt a "schlimazel" (in Yiddish: a person with chronic bad luck).

Driving with a wonky SOM requested to close my eye, hoping for the best.

I did not feel confident enough as to take the family in the car. My self-esteem was lower than the actual Titanic's waterline.

Despite being fully aware of the problems I was facing and my handicap, I used to be optimist getting into the car hoping to have a nice ride.

Unfortunately it did not last and things turned quite dangerous for every being into the vehicle and on the street.

So I faced the Jean Valjean dilemma: *"If I speak, I am condemned. If I stay silent, I am damned!"* And logically I could not help but feeling *misérable* for it.

I knew it was dangerous: if I avoided driving at all I got stalled at home if I kept doing it I put everyone in danger. And if I say something: who would support me? How would I keep my license?

All I can do was pulling the visors down blocking sunlight streaming, closing the eye to make a turn, identifying the actual image.

You feel unsafe driving to you, your passengers, the other vehicles and the poor pedestrian (AKA: easy targets).

Jerkiness is worse than duplicated vision since you can manage to recognize which image is the right one and do not get you as dazed as with a shaking vision.

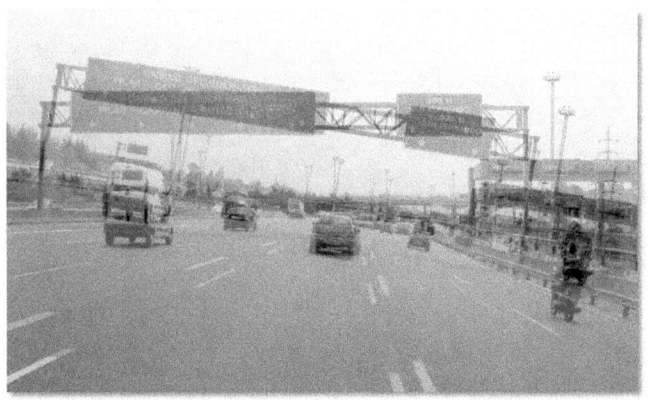

Picture 11: Dangerous driving.

A few times I had to pull over the car. Later I learned how to make a turn closing my twitchy eye.

At night, the lights of other cars affected me, not to mentions flash and intense lights of police cars, ambulances and fire trucks.

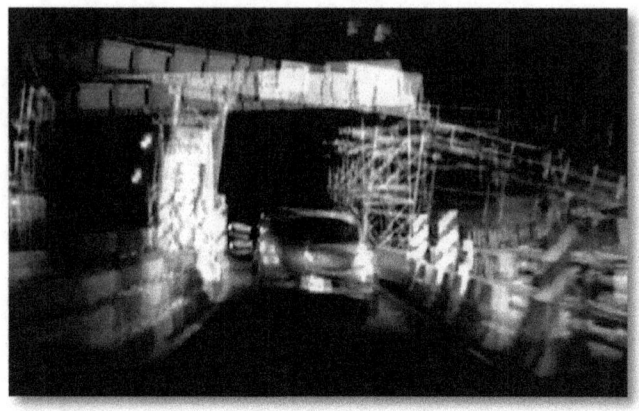

Picture 12: Driving at night.

Driving at night, could really drive you crazy.

Even in a good day the uncertainty of how long would it last until SOM plays up, kept me away from driving, What if I faint? What if I ended up crashed on the side of the road?

So I rarely dare to drive, and I got hopeless and embarrassed, being always seen on the front passenger seat.

Walking

Even walking was a challenge. I used to feel disoriented, stumbling and crashing into things.

To cross the street, since you cannot trust on your own senses, and a wonky eye damages the peripheral vision (the part of vision that occurs outside the very center of gaze).

So I had to do as in London streets: "look left, look right and look both sides", and sometimes more than once, and like a ritual, facing every single crosswalk.

This was particularly annoying since I had to turn the whole head, to check if a vehicle was coming, and it was safe to go ahead.

It was like the well-known Bigfoot picture. Have you seen it? The poor thing since –hypothetically- is not able to turn its face, has to turn its head along with its upper torso.

Looking both sides, meant to me turning my head. Not my face. Not my eyes. But the whole thing. Just like Bigfoot.

If I was OK, sometimes SOM was triggered if I looked at a certain angle, just as the new Windows 8 Hot Corners.

In my case, the bottom-left corner ran the shimmering, shaking, twisting, turning, and moving double vision program, so I had to avoid it.

When SOM was bothering me too much, in order to cross the street, when I turn my head, I had to wink or even cover my naughty eye.

Under that situation, the turning movement to look right and left, was not smooth at all, but it was kind of spasmodic. So it seemed I was virtually slapping myself in every corner!

If I focused at something, quickly shifting to another thing, especially to a distant or closer object, I got the fluttering symptoms.

Using the stairs could be dangerous. I had one episode of feeling dizzy and have to hold me to the handrail with both hands to avoid falling.

I noticed that I could not walk a straight line. It was not like staggering, but lightly straying to the left.

Biking

I got problems even riding my bike, but I also found that endorphins generated by the exercise helped a lot to counterweight SOM symptoms.

If you have a good SOMday, you can "commutercise" travelling to and from work by physical means (running, biking, skating, roller blading, etc.) instead of using mass transit or a car.

Truth is that I am not a sportsman. I just like, bicycling, walking and swimming.

Riding my bike was almost impossible. To the usual SOM confusion, the cycle tracks intermittently moved and got rudely doubled.

I found that maneuvering along the narrow bicycle lanes, especially when other bikes were around, was particularly difficult.

With SOM symptoms, walking was easiest thing to do. Broader sidewalks or parks were great to go outdoors. Dizziness existed, but at least without danger for me or other poor nearby souls.

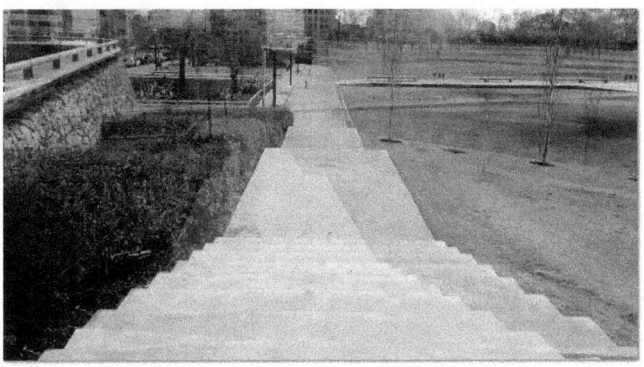

Picture 13: Go outdoors, just avoid the stairways!

GETTING OUT FROM THE FUNHOUSE TUNNEL

CHAPTER 6.
SOCIAL LIFE?

I am a stay-at-home person, but the truth is that facing the fact that I could not get out, I chose to think I made the decision to be alone at home, and do not pretend anymore.

I thought I decided to rather be alone.

Alright, let's face it: I used to keep to my home all the weekend because I simply was scared.

And even if I got out, I could not find a balance between being honest about my condition and whining all the time being a crying shame, so I ultimately stayed away from friends and rejected any invitation.

Why explain yourself? Paraphrasing Elbert Hubbard: "Never explain - your friends do not need it and your enemies will not believe you anyway."

Before SOM made me a better person, it made me a bitter one. I turned rancorous and harsh. I complaint all time. But did I complain about my eye? No, I had to pretend. So I complained about anything else.

Real friends perceive everything about you, and I had the privilege of counting on a few but very caring, courageous and sincere friends, who realized something was wrong before I even notice it.

Later I found that the topic I chose to whine about was, in fact, the main cause of my condition, but I was not able to recognize that fact that soon. Unfortunately, I had to wait for a louder call.

At a certain point, I was happy with everyone around me, but not happy with myself.

I did not realize all the things from which SOM was holding me back. I mean, shaving or even putting on my shoes was a chore.

Walking or moving stairways, was secretly huge for me. I would have a hard time even when doing nothing as long as I had my eyes opened.

But there is always a friend: someone willing to listen, someone willing to give advice, someone willing to warning us, and willing to reprehend us, and sometimes willing to get a better insight about how it is living with SOM.

Every aspect of my social life was disturbed by my condition, and the worse thing was that nobody truly understood my discomfort and pain.

Even those who supported me, I deeply knew, no matter how hard they tried; they did not fully comprehend how I was suffering.

I even suspected that most of them did not even believe me. At the time, I thought that it could be more credible, saying I had a close encounter of the Third Kind.

How to get people to know how SOM is

I purposefully got my eye irritated, to let the thin blood vessels of the eye got visible, and so I could record the eye movements on camera.

Thanks to the vessels as references, It was crystal clear the rotation of the eye on its own axis which otherwise could not be perceived.

I thought myself as an astronomer that find new planets, not by direct observation but based on the effect of its gravity and the distortion of the light.

I sent my video clip to the ophthalmologist, neuro-ophthalmologist and optometrist... and to my wife, father, mother, sister and mother-in-law..., and I was *this* close, to share it on all known social network (but that could be going too far).

This was the smoking gun, the objective evidence of my ailment. Not just an imaginary or intangible condition anymore.

I knew it did not deserve an Oscar nomination for a short film, but I was happy to catch this elusive thing on video.

But this only shows the movement of the eye, not how it looks from the SOMer perspective. How the heck you can show them how it feels having SOM without whining at all?

A picture is worth a thousand words. This was my low-cost trick:

I printed a picture of a face or a landscape in a regular paper and another copy of the very same image on a tracing paper.

I put both images together (the original on the back and the transparent ahead) and punched a hole in the bottom right corner.

I put a brass fastener through the hole and opened the leaves, or tines, of the legs, bent over to secure the paper.

This holds the pin in place and sheets of paper together. The split pin allows rotation around the joint.

And *voilà*! I got my own SOM simulator to illustrate the SOMer perception of the world!

My SOM caused a repetitive back and forth motion to upper-right corner; so I moved the tracing paper in a spasmodic vibration (or oscillation), around the joint, making it stop sometimes in the original place, and sometimes slightly twirled in such a way the image got duplicated slanting or inclined to the upper-right corner.

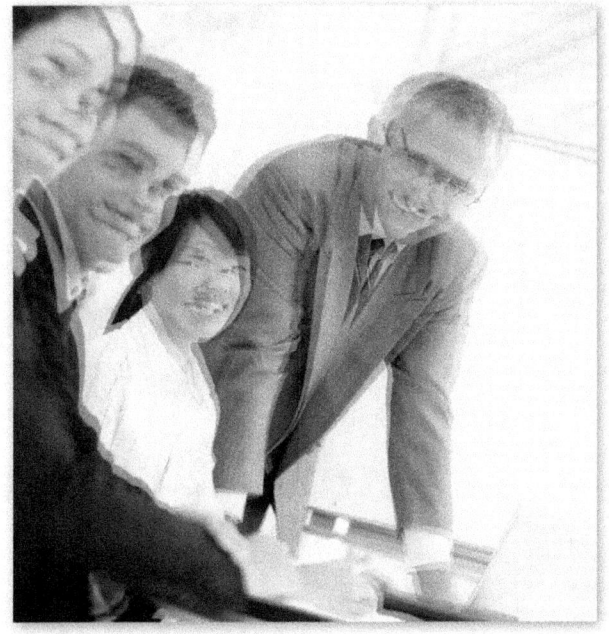

Picture 14: Each person had four eyes!

Then, people were able to understand how the SOM movement and double vision (diplopia) was.

You can customize it to fit your own experience and rotate it as quickly and spasmodically as your eye does.

I found this an extremely useful tool.

It clearly shows how it feels trying to make eye contact with a twister eye, which suddenly stops anywhere in the middle of its way –hopefully on its normal state- because if not, you see other people faces duplicated one image straight, and the other slightly tilted.

Vacations

One of the most uncomfortable experiences is when SOM joins you on your vacations.

You are expecting to relax, but sometimes the stress of the trip prevails and the symptoms continue.

Even "the happiest place on Earth" may seem quite gloomy.

Landmarks seem different from the picture of a souvenir shop's postcard.

If traveling to Italy –for instance- you would discover two coexisting versions of the leaning Tower of Pisa, one straight and the other leaning as people know it.

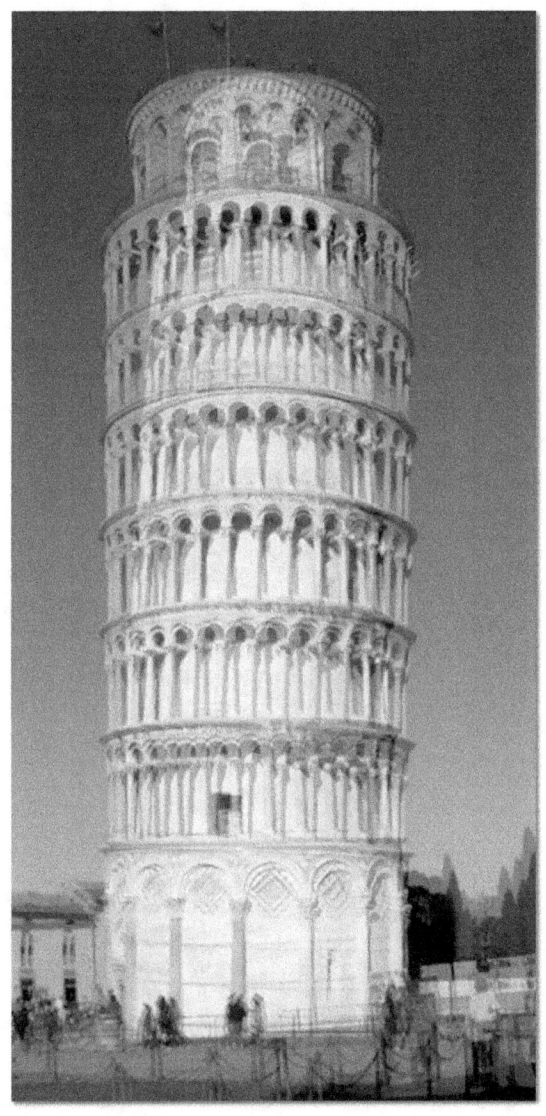

Picture 15: Lean and straight Pisa towers.

It takes time to get used to it, and to master the art of recognizing which is the image of the universe you belong to, and which one is the distorted illusion of the "parallel dimension of your mind".

Even if I wanted to hang out, how could I go?

Entertainment

Since you cannot drive, you cannot go to a concert, go to the theater or to a restaurant or vacationing by car wherever you want, whenever you want. You always depend on something or someone else, other person, public transportation or whatsoever.

Experiencing the movies:

I could not enjoy going to the movies as I used to love. Anyway, I went to see Avatar. Believe me, if Avatar 3D is a thing, you should see it in "Real SOM": that is THE ultimate experience. It becomes a theme park attraction created by a sadistic engineer!

Experiencing the theater:

A few years ago, for my birthday I was quite sad and my wife suggested we should go to the theater to see The New Mel Brooks Musical Young Frankenstein. I was resilient to go because it was a lot of money for a rather difficult SOMday.

But it was my birthday, and I agreed that the best thing would be to see something witty and funny. As we waited to get into the theater my eye was dreadful, and I did my best to handle it in place.

We sat down, the show began, I was controlling my SOM, and suddenly a strobe flashed straight to the audience (the last thing I needed) my eye went like crazy.

Experiencing the music:

"Music hath charms to soothe a savage breast, to soften rocks, or bend a knotted oak." William Congreve

* * *

One of the comforts I found to alleviate SOM was music.

As to tastes, nothing is written, but to me, one of the voices I like the most is Sarah Brightman's. Her music escorted me along the lengthy commuting hours.

Music tames the wild beast (and the most rebel eye). So many times I listened this music during relaxation exercises for my eye, that the relax sensation got linked to that music.

With time, just that voice could calm SOM down. It was taming a wild beast.

That is what NLP calls "anchoring" which means setting up an emotional response pattern triggered by something so that feeling can be prompted whenever it is needed it.

The rationale behind the decision to try this out, was the idea that if something could be a trigger that turn SOM on, then I could develop a trigger to turn it off.

Happily, it worked.

In 2009, Sarah Brightman came to Buenos Aires, and I decided to go no matter how my wild eye could behave.

After avoiding hanging out for so long, especially in jam-packed places, I was quite tense ... and so my eye.

The concert started. I closed my eyes decided to let myself go with the music... not just seeing a show, nor listening a song, but feeling with every sense, the music I love so deeply.

Then, I could say, was only time I thoroughly enjoyed music with every single sense. The tension faded away, and I could enjoyed the show.

When you cannot find your way out of the downward spiral caused by overwhelming stress and anguish, try turning to music.

Music can quickly shift your mood, altering the subconscious mind where pesky thoughts feed on your fears and fuel the fires of SOM.

Listening to music is inexpensive, quick-acting 24/7 solution, and it could just save your life.

Adding the music you like the most, engages more areas of the brain and can help you, over time, making us less susceptible to stress triggers.

Try to pick those with positive lyrics, it will work as a mantra. The repetition of music, can be a great technique to turn to whenever you start to feel stressed or overwhelmed.

Accompanied by your clear intention, you will be able to get a joyful state. The more emotion and the greater the number of repetitions the stronger the effect will be.

The fact is that no matter what music you like the most, or causes the same effect, rock, techno, rap or whatsoever, you can "train" your eye to be relaxed with a musical trigger.

PART II:
GETTING OUT FROM THE
FUNHOUSE TUNNEL

CHAPTER 7.
GAME OVER

February 2nd, 2012. I thought I was dying...

That summer morning I woke up extremely early.

I had to get at work earlier to achieve the inconsequential goal of pleasing my boss.

It was hot even at 5 AM. I walked to the bus stop as usual, except that it was early in the morning, and I was already sweated.

Buses were so full they did not stop. I had to wait 40 minutes to get into one. During the waiting, as the sun rose just on my face, SOM symptoms were already extremely intense.

The bus ride was worse than ever, a cattle truck could have been more comfortable.

On the way, the bus stopped at the railroad crossing. The gate arms were down for half an hour in advance until the train finally passed.

The sun through the bus window made kind of greenhouse effect and the sun glare right at my face worsen the bumping vision, and I was getting grumpy minding my own business.

The bus continued its road. Later, even I rang the bell in advance, the driver skipped the bus stop where I had to get off (he clearly was in a hurry too and wanted to take advantage of the green traffic light).

I got off the bus and ran those extra blocks to the subway station. Downstairs, the cardboard sign over the turnstile gate indicated that the subway service was delayed –once more.

A multitude waited, overcrowding the unique platform that is used both for departures as arrivals.

Being on the platform, you do not know whether the train will come or leave from the right or left track; it is totally random.

However after more than 1,440 trips departing from that station; I realized that if no subway is already on the station, statistically in 80% of the cases, it stops on the left and leave first, so I did my bet accordingly. I was hoping to have some chance to get a seat or choose a convenient spot to be standing.

Well, it came from the right.

I was pushed by the crowd into the subway car ending up in its hottest corner.

As the hot aged subway raced my mind started to spin around, questioning if all the effort I have been doing to succeed –including the daily rides- really worth it.

The subway spent a lot more than usual on each stop and even stopped in the gap between stations.

It was not even close to the last station (where I had to get off) and the sweat to get early to my job, already turned out to be worthless.

Racing thoughts whirled in my mind as the screeching subway noise blended with the cursing of rude people that complained out loud about everything; blaming the politician they detested the most for the second-rate transportation service.

Hostility arose as people argued, pushed and called one to each other every name under the sun.

The foul air was not breathable, and I started to take faster and shorter breaths.

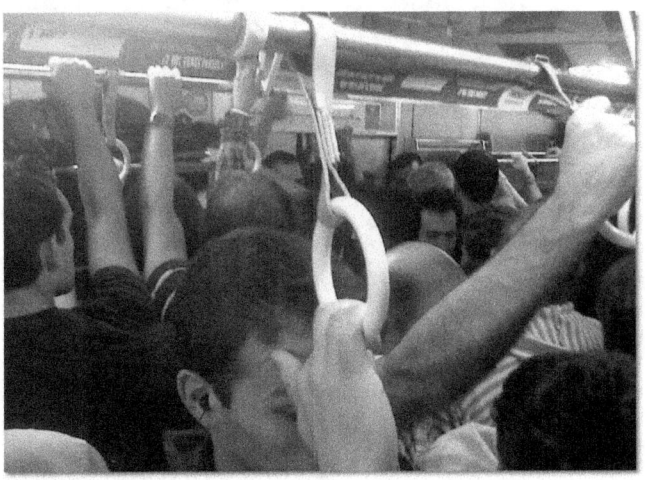

Picture 16: Subway: another day in paradise...

Even not the stinky hot wind that came through the windows –which happens to be the only acclimatizing system- could ease the extreme heat.

My mind was in high gear, while questioning to myself a lot of things, and my eye was going extremely wild.

A swarm of sticky passengers pushed one to another, as my jerking eye made a funhouse tunnel out of the subway car.

The whole thing violently whirled around me. It was hard to remain calm and safe from that dense atmosphere.

The subway reached the final station.

The throng pushed forward to get the exit bursting out the car like a water pressure relief in a damn, leaving the car empty except of me, that remained way behind the multitude.

I was stepping out of the car already sick, and then, alone, just crossing the gap between the car and the platform, my bumping vision got blurry.

Tired of pretending that everything was OK, to fight against the constant tremors of my sight and overwhelmed by stress, I built up to a nervous breakdown.

Totally overburdened, I was finally borne down by adversity, and I felt fainting.

I did not lose consciousness, but I felt I was going to. I started feeling a rapid heartbeat.

Terrified I reached the escalator with one single thought in mind: "I cannot die here".

I was clinging at the escalator handrail, and as soon I got to the first level, I asked for help to the subway guard and the ambulance came.

I finally knuckled under to the pressure.

I was took by an ambulance, and since my wife was taking care of my kids, as humiliating as it may sound, I had no choice but to call my mother.

The first thing I told her was "I thought I was dying", the second one was "I do not remember when was the last time I saw something without SOM, anymore".

...I will hold the following embarrassing emotional reactions to myself.

Later on, I had a comprehensive medical check-up, and happily, everything was OK.

Once I calm down I told the doctor: "people say that when dying, your life flashes before your eyes like a fast-forward movie; I am just 39 and I saw my whole life before my eyes but it was so short it was not even close to a f* teaser trailer!"

The Doc said I was lucky. That my body talked to me, so I had to work on paying attention to those callings and manage the emotions which were linked to hypertension and the Panic Attacks (which, by the way, never returned).

If he said that my body talked to me, and there was an obvious connection between Panic Attacks and hypertension, could it be possible that my long lasting SOM was a constant wake-up call?

SOM was the first thing I could notice before everything else skyrocketed.

Some part of me actually died right there and then, getting ready for something brand new. I have past the point of no return already.

Could I get something good out of it? Was this episode a blessing in disguise?

It was something like this indeed, not because of its intrinsic nature (it was awful), but rather because I chose to change the way I saw it.

It was not easy. It was not immediate.

I took five months of sabbaticals dedicated exclusively to resolve my condition.

It was an extremely demanding work of learning and unlearning, testing and failing, questioning and answering, just to question everything all again.

One day, I was walking when I realized that something very strange was going on. Something different... I suddenly noticed the difference "Everything is so quiet! –I thought".

At last, I was SOMless for a long time!

I was so programmed to be on guard against SOM that I had not realized it was fading away.

As I went through that healing journey, SOMless moments became days, weeks and months, and SOM symptoms have been gradually vanishing.

I tried very hard not to think about the possibility or probability of any remission. I tried hard to completely remove that kind of thinking.

At first, I felt as I were fearful walking on a tightrope. Everything was a threat. Any wrong decision or inconvenience any thought could get me off balance and would fall –again- to the depths of SOM.

I was troubled thinking about what would happen to me when I return to work.

The situation of the business became more complicated than ever, because of the economy turndown and domestic political issues, so everything was nothing but uncertainties for everyone.

But I returned. Stronger and I could face every challenge that was presented with assertiveness.

I used to think that my come back would be gradual, you know, something like the NASA's probe "Deep Space One" which each day adds about 20 mph its speed getting after 300 days 60,000 (mph).

But it was not anything like that, but as one of its rocket launch, requiring all its power from the very first moment.

It was rough, it was interminable, but I made it. I was finally back, and 100% SOMfree.

CHAPTER 8.
"VINI, VIDI, VICI" (I CAME, I SAW, I SUCCEED)

"Your visions will become clear only when you can look into your own heart. Who looks outside, dreams; who looks inside, awakes." — C.G. Jung

* * *

It has been more than a year without SOM, or better said with SOM as an instrument at my service, with no symptoms that neither restrict my activities nor confine myself.

I can assert that I came into the funhouse tunnel, I saw it, and I succeed (getting out from it).

And as a lesson learned I am entitled to sustain that the most difficult thing to start with, is finding someone that honestly could say:

I DO UNDERSTAND YOU.

I think that medicine does not heal, but helps the body heal itself. I do not intend to heal your SOM through this book neither.

My intention is more humble: bringing to you some comfort and that necessary condition of being truly understood, to let you find your way out from the funhouse tunnel.

Getting the whole picture

OK, enough whining already. I do not want it, and you do not need it.

Once you know you have SOM, it is complete pointless to research the anatomical and functional source of it. Let the doctors do their work.

You have to work on a more urgent work: focusing on getting yourself out from the funhouse tunnel that SOM means to you.

You are entitled to claim your quality of life back.

An exclusively ophthalmic approximation is – ironically- rather shortsighted in order to figure out how to overcome SOM.

A holistic approach is needed to succeed. Hypertension, Panic Attack, SOM and other stress-related pathologies such as dandruff, dermatitis and irritable bowel syndrome seem to be somehow associated.

Even the correlation is not proven by science you can find it by your own, with an attentive and rational reflection of your symptoms and its context.

Between the SOM triggers and its symptoms there is a space and time. A context that no matter how short it could be, should be used to relax, think and see how do you feel, and why are you feeling that way.

Understanding your SOM will lead to a better understanding of yourself.

Quicksand analogy

SOM is like quicksand that keep you trapped. However, there are seven steps to get people out from there. I realized this could fit your situation like if you find yourself in quicksand:

Step 1. Leave out everything.

Since your body is less dense than quicksand, you cannot fully sink unless you panic and struggle or you are weighed down by something heavy. I found that the best way to get rid of SOM was learning to get along with it, because just like if you step into quicksand, the more you fight it, the more difficult it is to get out of it.

You immediately should take off your backpack full of fears and any idea that restricts you to prevail. Unlearn the concept, that something is incurable or should last forever.

The mere idea of something impossible makes nonsense. It used to be impossible to reach the moon, and there is a flag there already, it used to be impossible to let deaf people hear, and now it is possible.

The simple fact that the answer is still unknown does not mean there is no answer. Give science the time it needs, but do not take for granted labels.

If you have your diagnostic made by a professional, let it be. Keep yourself positive sure it is SOM and nothing more. Do not let your mind ever think it could possibly be another thing or get worse. Sweep away any negative thought about the situation and about yourself. Leave any judgment about yourself. SOM is not a punishment or a weakness. Let other conditions and fears out of the scene. Do not act as an hypochondriac.

As I mentioned before, I used to be an hypochondriac. That aspect of my personality did not leave me alone and used to bring to my mind every possible fear about SOM.

I was sure that in order to get rid of SOM, I first should get rid of this hypochondriac inside me. So I thought that I should create something easy, practical and nice (remember, in order to succeed, you have to avoid any negative thought, so fight against yourself is just pointless).

So I asked myself "who is the worst hypochondriac person I know of? –and Woody Allen came to my mind."

From that moment on, every time I single fearful thought came to my mind, I said to myself : "Go away Woody." It was not a joke. It was not something I did once. It was an friendly order I gave every single time.

And the seemingly stupid fact of putting a name for it was essential. Giving an order to another person, does not end up as an aggressive intimidation against yourself, I kept myself and accept myself avoiding any kind of judgment.

Leave your back bag behind, remember?

Get out of the relationships that, as boots, hold you in the quicksand and pull you down even deeper.

Do not accept, by any means, substandard nor asymmetrical relationships. For substandard, I mean those relationships or conditions you do not deserve. For asymmetrical, I mean those relationships or conditions that force you to give more than you get, no matter if it is money, recognition, loyalty or satisfaction.

Step 2. Relax.

SOM could be just a light discomfort, a shallow swamp. Even if you experience across an extremely strong SOM, you could very well sink no more than your waist or chest, but if you panic you can sink further. So take it easy, your body's buoyancy will keep you safe right there. Calm down, and your new attitude and mindset will prevent you to fall into a more serious SOM experience.

Step 3. Breathe.

Deep breathing will help you stay calm, but it also lets you be more buoyant. It is not possible to be submerged if you have air in your lungs.

Breathing is instrumental to relaxation, but it is also an end by itself. Visualize in your mind that, in every breath, you send air to your eye (I do know it sound strange, but it worked for me).

Step 4. Get on your back.

If you sink up to your hips bend backward. That position requires a lot of self-confidence, and that is the idea. You can manage your SOM. Use your own confidence, strengths and capabilities on every aspect of your life.

This is like distributing your weight, to preventing you to sink. While floating on your back, working on every aspect of your life, you will prudently release your legs and then can inch yourself to safety smoothly propelling yourself to the edge.

Step 5. Take your time.

If you are in quicksand, frantic movements will be futile. To get off your SOM, whatever you do, do it at a snail's pace. As agitating the quicksand; vibrations cause firm ground into more quicksand, energetic behaviors may worsen your condition or the right atmosphere to get effective results.

Since there is trial and error to self-discover your way out, you have to go slowly paying attention to the reaction methodically and patiently.

And when I say patiently, I mean it. I –as most of us- was raised on a fast-food culture where everything should be immediate.

Well, let's put it this way: In order to get rid of SOM, I had to learn to see the rocks grow.

Step 6. Take regular breaks.

Getting out of quicksand could be quite a long journey, take breaks floating on your back. Go baby steps, and take some time off.

You will be working on yourself, and as any work, there is some tension. Release that stress planning or improvising pauses.

Step 7. Use a stick.

A stick and some maneuvers can be helpful to getting you out from quicksand. Your stick may be your partner, a relative, a friend or a medical practitioner, psychologist, counselor or any professional you have confidence.

As a stick, you should "use" these people brainy. Everyone should have a specific role. You cannot cry a river over everyone or cling over every shoulder.

You have to make your relationships work for you and protect these relationships, avoiding conflicts and the expected wear and tear.

It is a matter of counting on people to help you, avoiding consuming those relationships along the way.

These seven steps, can help you out, in the short term, to build and strengthen your attitude, capabilities, relationships and environment for a quick recovery of your life quality.

Quality of life

"I am the master of my fate: I am the captain of my soul" -William Ernest Henley (b. August 23rd, 1849)

* * *

It had been such a long time since the last time I drove! I could not believe I was driving again! First just a few blocks away from home (those you know as yourself) and later, a little further and the more I did it, the more confident I became.

Sometime later, I was able to take my children to their school and to the movies and to the park, and then I dare to take the family for a weekend out from the city driving in a highway. I was so excited!

Not to mention when I ventured to drive at night with my family! I had forgotten how it feels.

My kids have never experienced how was traveling at night, they were so thrilled.

"Look dad! How many lights!" -They said as country kids visiting the big city for their first time.

I was proudly in charge of the steering wheel of my life again.

I taught my kids to ride their bikes without helping wheels, and it was so important to me, it was an emotional memory as I know they will not ever forget it, and neither I.

From that moment on, riding our bikes together remains me all I had to go through to make it happen.

And it also makes me wonder: would I have given that moment the value it actually had, if I would not have to go through this affliction.

All those nights of panic and trembling sight, where I hold my kids with my eyes closed until they fall asleep, striving to discern the subtlest smell of their hair because I had to keep my eyes shut.

Gosh! I did not realize my son still smelt like a baby or the soft cheek of my daughter when I used to kiss her goodnight!

Everything used to be so conditioned to the visual sense.

After all this experience, when they ask me "what are you doing?" I am still responding: "I am enjoying!"

You should provide yourself some satisfaction, some pleasure and enjoyment. It could be a physical, intellectual or emotional gratification.

I was enjoying so many things again, but at the same time, enjoying in a different way as I became aware more sensitive of other features and feelings beside the visual characteristic and stimulus.

Was this learning necessary to understand what I already knew? I think it was.

There certainly are magnificent scents, flavors, sounds, textures and feelings, all hidden by sight, invisible, behind the domain of an invincible and frantic visual reign, patiently waiting to be revealed and enjoyed.

SOM is a pain, but it also an opportunity to let you discover this kind of little things.

* * *

"Recently I was visited by a very good friend who had just returned from a long walk in the woods, and I asked her what she had observed. "Nothing in particular," she replied. I might have been incredulous had I not been accustomed to such responses, for long ago I became convinced that the seeing see little. How was it possible, I asked myself, to walk for an hour through the woods and see nothing worthy of note? I who cannot see find hundreds of things to interest me through mere touch. I feel the delicate symmetry of a leaf. I pass my hands lovingly about the smooth skin of a silver birch, or the rough, shaggy bark of a pine. In spring, I touch the branches of trees hopefully in search of a bud, the first sign of awakening Nature after her winter's sleep. I feel the delightful, velvety texture of a flower, and discover its remarkable convolutions, and something of the miracle of Nature is revealed to me."
-Helen Keller. Three Days to See (1933)

Do you know what I mean?

With a little help of my friends

I told you: it was not a mere metaphysical journey. I wish it were!

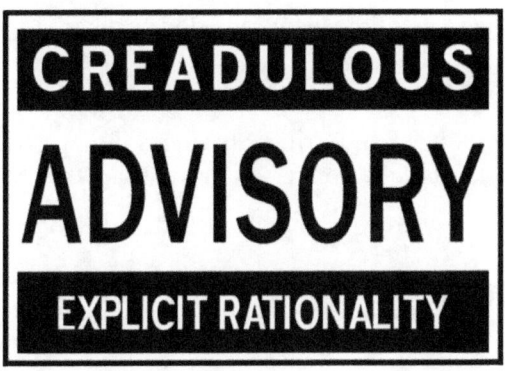

As part of this open chronicle, I have to admit that due to the intense shock caused by the episode in the subway, at the begging, I was medicated with a mood stabilizer.

This is something I have never been excited or pleased for. I did not want to accept it nor disclose it beyond my closest circle.

I just did not like it, but I only accepted it to boost the recovery and then drop it as soon as possible.

I was reluctant about the dependence that it may induce (if any) and the trouble of being stigmatized as a weak person or sickly worker (which I am certainly not).

Medication was meant to help me to go through that situation more effectively, and it certainly did.

I did not get to the point where it would be necessary to visit GAP looking for the trendiest straitjacket, but –I told you it was hard- every now and then I had one of those ups and downs days.

* * *

After a week of terrible SOMdays, I met a friend at Starbucks, and the conversation went like this:

- How are you going? –asked my friend.

- Well depends on the day –I said. I have those days when it's impossible to stand my eye problem and I am sad, angry and negative.

- It sound terrible. Is every day like that?

- Of course not! Those are my good days!

* * *

It happens that the prescribed medication I was taking, is used in the treatment of mood disorders (that was good) and –at the same time- as anticonvulsants (that was very good).

Anticonvulsants are some drugs that were originally used in epilepsy patients, but science quickly discovered its effectiveness in the treatment of mood disorders.

Even though SOM effects were already fading away, this treatment certainly seemed to be useful to speed up the healing process.

In my case, it was indicated Alprazolam which is prescribed for the treatment of generalized anxiety disorder and Panic Attacks.

Lamotrigine also applied. It is a drug, used especially for epilepsy, and bipolar disorder. Lamotrigine is used, primarily, for the treatment of epilepsy and also as a mood stabilizer.

As funny as it seems, how Lamotrigine works is still unknown, but it did for me, and it has fewer side effects than other drugs.

With the help of a professional, I took advantage of these medications, which were gradually reduced and yet the SOM did not recur as ferocious as it used to be.

Believe me, taking so many different pills that an M&M bag seemed monochromatic was no funny at all and completely different from a new age-ish and one-size-fits-all solution.

Later on, I understood that I was able to handle stress in such a way that I did not need medication at the same extent.

In the late episodes, facing SOM symptoms, I paid attention and noticed I was in pain for a contracture of my back muscles; so I simply took a non-prescription pain reliever, which are particularly effective to reduce muscle soreness.

Once I set free from pain, with some relaxation and –if possible a short walking outdoors- the symptoms faded away.

So I can attest that medication helped, but it was not the only factor –the silver bullet.

Medicine worked for what it was meant to do, as long as I became more self-confident of my ability to control SOM and learned how to deal with stress in a more efficient way.

I was ready and got in a mood, suitable to learn about breathing, mindfulness and how to control reactions that I once thought were unchangeable.

With peace of mind, I turned to be a more flexible, tolerant, composed and assertive person. Not that I am the Dalai Lama or someone like him. I am not in a Nirvana the whole day or anything like that, but at least I can control myself responding to situations, but not impulsively reacting at them, as I used to.

If something bothered me, I was able to think "what is happening here?". When I could not do it, my eye asked it for myself (and let me know about that, with its usual manners).

I soon realized that I rather play it easy, and ask any question myself.

Other useful medication that helped me the overnight relief of the eye was a Soothe Night Time Lubricant Eye Ointment.

I mentioned it in previous chapters. It is like a gel. It helped me to feel more relaxed in the morning, and so SOM used to get significantly eased.

CHAPTER 9.
STRESS MANAGEMENT

"Stress is when you wake up screaming and you realize you haven't even fallen asleep yet."

* * *

The reason I added this chapter is because I found that stress is really a powder keg for SOM.

This is not a Stress Management book, but if you read the previous chapter, you will understand how important this issue is for people forced to live with SOM.

Let me tell you this. At first I was skeptical. I was so immerse in my own problems, I did not realize of the stress I was amassing.

The first readings about this matter, I was like: "Duh! I have a problem here, give me some answers. I need some practical quick-win solutions." I mean, the first time I heard about that there are two kind of stress:

the well-known bad one, and the good one, my reaction was like someone would have told me that there is a bad diarrhea and a good one (I am sorry for the scatological reference).

While we are all under stress at times, our bodies react in different ways and SOM is one sign of stress. Reducing the cause of the stress can help you make SOM stop.

Along the following sections, I will share with you the key element of Stress Management that I found useful to manage SOM.

I know you are going to be able to associate the next information, with my own experience, and get a better understanding of it, as well as get some practical tips you could apply in your own situation.

Stress Symptoms, Signs, & Causes: The Effects of Stress Overload and What You Can Do About It

Modern life is full of hassles, deadlines, frustrations, and demands. For many people, stress is so commonplace that it has become a way of life. Stress is not always bad. In small doses, it can help you perform under pressure and motivate you to do your best. But when you are constantly running in emergency mode, your mind and body pay the price. You can protect yourself by recognizing the signs and symptoms of stress and taking steps to reduce its harmful effects.

What is stress?

Stress is a normal physical response to events that make you feel threatened or upset your balance in some way. When you sense danger—whether it's real or imagined—the body's defenses kick into high gear in a rapid, automatic process known as the "fight-or-flight-or-freeze" reaction, or the stress response.

The stress response is the body's way of protecting you. When working properly, it helps you stay focused, energetic, and alert. In emergency situations, stress can save your life—giving you extra strength to defend yourself, for example, or spurring you to slam on the brakes to avoid an accident.

The stress response also helps you rise to meet challenges. Stress is what keeps you on your toes during a presentation at work, sharpens your concentration when you are attempting the game-winning free throw, or drives you to study for an exam when you'd rather be watching TV.

But beyond a certain point, stress stops being helpful and starts causing major damage to your health, your mood, your productivity, your relationships, and your quality of life.

The Body's Stress Response

When you perceive a threat, your nervous system responds by releasing a flood of stress hormones, including adrenaline and cortisol. These hormones rouse the body for emergency action.

Your heart pounds faster, muscles tighten, blood pressure rises, breath quickens, and your senses become sharper. These physical changes increase your strength and stamina, speed your reaction time, and enhance your focus—preparing you to either fight or flee from the danger at hand.

How do you respond to stress?

It's important to learn how to recognize when your stress levels are out of control. The most dangerous thing about stress is how easily it can creep up on you. You get used to it. It starts to feel familiar, even normal. You don't notice how much it's affecting you, even as it takes a heavy toll.

The signs and symptoms of stress overload can be almost anything. Stress affects the mind, body, and behavior in many ways, and everyone experiences stress differently. Not only can overwhelming stress lead to serious mental and physical health problems, it can also take a toll on your relationships at home, work, and school.

Stress doesn't always look stressful

Psychologist Connie Lillas uses a driving analogy to describe the three most common ways people respond when they are overwhelmed by stress:

* Foot on the gas – An angry, agitated, or "fight" stress response. you are heated, keyed up, overly emotional, and unable to sit still.

* Foot on the brake – A withdrawn, depressed, or "flight" stress response. You shutdown, pull away, space out, and show very little energy or emotion.

* Foot on both – A tense or "freeze" stress response. You become frozen under

pressure and can't do anything. You look paralyzed, but under the surface you are extremely agitated.

Signs and symptoms of stress overload

The following table lists some of the common warning signs and symptoms of stress. The more signs and symptoms you notice in yourself, the closer you may be to stress overload.

Cognitive Symptoms

* Memory problems

* Inability to concentrate

* Poor judgment

* Seeing only the negative

* Anxious or racing thoughts

* Constant worrying

Emotional Symptoms

* Moodiness

* Irritability or short temper

* Agitation, inability to relax

* Feeling overwhelmed

* Sense of loneliness and isolation

* Depression or general unhappiness

Physical Symptoms

* Aches and pains

* Diarrhea or constipation

* Nausea, dizziness

* Chest pain, rapid heartbeat

* Loss of sex drive

* Frequent colds

Behavioral Symptoms

* Eating more or less

* Sleeping too much or too little

* Isolating yourself from others

* Procrastinating or neglecting responsibilities

* Using alcohol, cigarettes, or drugs to relax

* Nervous habits (e.g. nail biting, pacing)

Keep in mind that the signs and symptoms of stress can also be caused by other psychological or medical problems. If you are experiencing any of the warning signs of stress, it's important to see a doctor for a full evaluation. Your doctor can help you determine whether or not your symptoms are stress-related.

How much stress is too much?

Because of the widespread damage stress can cause, it's important to know your own limit. But just how much stress is "too much" differs from person to person. we are all different. Some people are able to roll with the punches, while others seem to crumble in the face of far smaller obstacles or frustrations. Some people even seem to thrive on the excitement and challenge of a high-stress lifestyle.

Your ability to tolerate stress depends on many factors, including the quality of your relationships, your general outlook on life, your emotional intelligence, and genetics.

Things that influence your stress tolerance level

* Your support network – A strong network of supportive friends and family members can be an enormous buffer against life's stressors. On the flip side, the more lonely and isolated you are, the greater your vulnerability to stress.

* Your sense of control – It may be easier to take stress in your stride if you have confidence in yourself and your ability to influence events and persevere through challenges. If you feel like things are out of your control, you are likely to have less tolerance for stress.

* Your attitude and outlook – Optimistic people are often more stress-hardy. They tend to embrace challenges, have a strong sense of humor, and accept that change is a part of life.

* Your ability to deal with your emotions – you are extremely vulnerable to stress if you don't know how to calm and soothe yourself when you are feeling sad, angry, or overwhelmed by a situation. The ability to bring your emotions into balance helps you bounceback from adversity and is a skill that can be learned at any age.

*   Your knowledge and preparation – The more you know about a stressful situation, including how long it will last and what to expect, the easier it is to cope. For example, if you go into surgery with a realistic picture of what to expect post-op, a painful recovery will be less traumatic than if you were expecting to bounce back immediately.

Causes of stress

The situations and pressures that cause stress are known as stressors. We usually think of stressors as being negative, such as an exhausting work schedule or a rocky relationship. However, anything that puts high demands on you or forces you to adjust can be stressful. This includes positive events such as getting married, buying a house, going to college, or receiving a promotion.

Of course, not all stress is caused by external factors. Stress can also be self-generated, for example, when you worry excessively about something that may or may not happen, or have irrational, pessimistic thoughts about life.

What causes stress depends, at least in part, on your perception of it. Something that's stressful to you may not faze someone else; they may even enjoy it. For example, your morning commute may make you anxious and tense because you worry that traffic will make you late. Others, however, may find the trip relaxing because they allow more than enough time and enjoy listening to music while they drive.

Common external causes of stress

* Major life changes

* Work or school

* Relationship difficulties

* Financial problems

* Being too busy

* Children and family

Common internal causes of stress

* Chronic worry

* Pessimism

* Negative self-talk

* Unrealistic expectations/Perfectionism

* Rigid thinking, lack of flexibility

* All-or-nothing attitude

Effects of chronic stress

The body doesn't distinguish between physical and psychological threats. When you are stressed over a busy schedule, an argument with a friend, a traffic jam, or a mountain of bills, your body reacts just as strongly as if you were facing a life-or-death situation. If you have a lot of responsibilities and worries, your emergency stress response may be "on" most of the time. The more your body's stress system is activated, the harder it is to shut off.

Long-term exposure to stress can lead to serious health problems. Chronic stress disrupts nearly every system in your body. It can raise blood pressure, suppress the immune system, increase the risk of heart attack and stroke, contribute to infertility, and speed up the aging process. Long-term stress can even rewire the brain, leaving you more vulnerable to anxiety and depression.

Many health problems are caused or exacerbated by stress, including:

* Pain of any kind

* Heart disease

* Digestive problems

* Sleep problems

* Depression

* Weight problems

* Autoimmune diseases

* Skin conditions, such as eczema

Dealing with stress and its symptoms

While unchecked stress is undeniably damaging, you have more control over your stress levels than you might think. Unfortunately, many people cope with stress in ways that only compound the problem. You might drink too much to unwind at the end of a stressful day, fill up on comfort food, zone out in front of the TV or computer for hours, use pills to relax, or relieve stress by lashing out at other people. However, there are many healthier ways to cope with stress and its symptoms.

Since everyone has a unique response to stress, there is no "one size fits all" solution to dealing with it. No single method works for everyone or in every situation, so experiment with different techniques and strategies. Focus on what makes you feel calm and in control.

Learn how to manage stress

You may feel like the stress in your life is out of your control, but you can always control the way you respond. Managing stress is all about taking charge: taking charge of your thoughts, your emotions, your schedule, your environment, and the way you deal with problems. Stress management involves changing the stressful situation when you can, changing your reaction when you can't, taking care of yourself, and making time for rest and relaxation.

Remember the four As: avoid, alter, adapt, or accept.

* Avoid unnecessary stress. Not all stress can be avoided, but by learning how to say no, distinguishing between "shoulds" and "musts" on your to-do list, and steering clear of people or situations that stress you out, you can eliminate many daily stressors.

* Alter the situation. If you can't avoid a stressful situation, try to alter it. Be more assertive and deal with problems head on. Instead of bottling up your feelings and increasing your stress, respectfully let others know about your concerns. Or be more willing to compromise and try meeting others halfway on an issue.

* Adapt to the stressor. When you can't change the stressor, try changing yourself.

Reframe problems or focus on the positive things in your life. If a task at work has you stressed, focus on the aspects of your job you do enjoy. And always look at the big picture: is this really something worth getting upset about?

* Accept the things you can't change. There will always be stressors in life that you can't do anything about. Learn to accept the inevitable rather than rail against a situation and making it even more stressful. Look for the upside in a situation—even the most stressful circumstances can be an opportunity for learning or personal growth. Learn to accept that no one, including you, is ever perfect.

You can also better cope with the symptoms of stress by strengthening your physical health.

* Set aside relaxation time. Relaxation techniques such as yoga, meditation, and deep breathing activate the body's relaxation response, a state of restfulness that is the opposite of the stress response.

* Exercise regularly. Physical activity plays a key role in reducing and preventing the effects of stress. Nothing beats aerobic exercise for releasing pent-up stress and tension.

* Eat a healthy diet. Well-nourished bodies are better prepared to cope with stress. Start your day with a healthy breakfast, reduce your caffeine and sugar intake, and cut back on alcohol and nicotine.

* Get plenty of sleep. Feeling tired can increase stress by causing you to think irrationally. Keep your cool by getting a good night's sleep.

Take a 5-step program to relieve stress and bring your life into balance

Sometimes stress management is not enough. If you feel overwhelmed by stress but can't seem to follow through with a stress management program, you may need extra help. Helpguide's free online program can help you relieve stress and replace old emotional habits with healthier ways of thinking, feeling, behaving, and relating to others.

As well as learning why emotional intelligence is so important to your physical and emotional health, you'll also learn two core skills for reducing overwhelming stress: quick stress relief and emotional connection.

* Quick stress relief. The best way to reduce stress quickly and reliably is by using your senses—what you see, hear, smell, taste, and touch—or through movement. By viewing a favorite photo, smelling a specific scent, listening to a favorite piece of music, tasting a piece of gum, or hugging a pet, for example, you can quickly relax and focus yourself. Of course, not everyone responds to each sensory experience in the

same way. Something that relaxes one person may do nothing but irritate someone else. The key is to experiment with your senses and discover the sensory experiences that work best for you.

* Emotional connection. Nothing contributes more to chronic stress than emotional disconnection from ourselves and others. Understanding the influence emotions have on your thoughts and actions is vital to managing stress. Life doesn't have to feel like a rollercoaster ride with extreme ups and downs. Once you are aware of your emotions, even the painful ones you normally try to avoid or bottle up, the easier it is to understand your own motivations, stop saying or doing things you later regret, gain renewed energy, and smooth out the ride.

Once you've mastered these core skills you'll have the confidence to face stressful challenges, knowing that you'll always be able to rapidly bring yourself back into balance.

Stress at work: tips

While some workplace stress is normal, excessive stress can interfere with your productivity and impact your physical and emotional health. And your ability to deal with it can mean the difference between success or failure.

You can't control everything in your work environment, but that doesn't mean you are powerless—even when you are stuck in a difficult situation. Finding ways to manage workplace stress is not about making huge changes or rethinking career ambitions, but rather about focusing on the one thing that's always within your control: you.

Coping with work stress in today's uncertain climate

For workers everywhere, the troubled economy may feel like an emotional roller coaster. "Layoffs" and "budget cuts" have become bywords in the workplace, and the result is increased fear, uncertainty, and higher levels of stress. Since job and workplace stress increase in times of economic crisis, it's important to learn new and better ways of coping with the pressure.

Your emotions are contagious, and stress has an impact on the quality of your interactions with others. The better you are at managing your own stress, the more you'll positively affect those around you, and the less other people's stress will negatively affect you.

You can learn how to manage job stress

There are a variety of steps you can take to reduce both your overall stress levels and the stress you find on the job and in the workplace. These include:

* Taking responsibility for improving your physical and emotional well-being.

* Avoiding pitfalls by identifying knee jerk habits and negative attitudes that add to the stress you experience at work.

* Learning better communication skills to ease and improve your relationships with management and coworkers.

Tip 1: Recognize warning signs of excessive stress at work

When you feel overwhelmed at work, you lose confidence and may become irritable or withdrawn. This can make you less productive and less effective in your job, and make the work seem less rewarding. If you ignore the warning signs of work stress, they can lead to bigger problems. Beyond interfering with job performance and satisfaction, chronic or intense stress can also lead to physical and emotional health problems.

Signs and symptoms of excessive job and workplace stress

* Feeling anxious, irritable, or depressed

* Apathy, loss of interest in work

* Problems sleeping

* Fatigue

* Trouble concentrating

* Muscle tension or headaches

* Stomach problems

* Social withdrawal

* Loss of sex drive

* Using alcohol or drugs to cope

Common causes of excessive workplace stress

* Fear of being laid off

* More overtime due to staff cutbacks

* Pressure to perform to meet rising expectations but with no increase in job satisfaction

* Pressure to work at optimum levels—all the time!

Tip 2: Reduce job stress by taking care of yourself

When stress at work interferes with your ability to perform in your job, manage your personal life, or adversely impacts your health, it's time to take action. Start by paying attention to your physical and emotional health. When your own needs are taken care of, you are stronger and more resilient to stress. The better you feel, the better equipped you'll be to manage work stress without becoming overwhelmed.

Taking care of yourself doesn't require a total lifestyle overhaul. Even small things can lift your mood, increase your energy, and make you feel like you are back in the driver's seat. Take things one step at a time, and as you make more positive lifestyle choices, you'll soon notice a reduction in your stress levels, both at home and at work.

Get moving

Regular exercise is a powerful stress reliever—even though it may be the last thing you feel like doing. Aerobic exercise—activity that raises your heart rate and makes you sweat—is a hugely effective way to lift your mood, increase energy, sharpen focus, and relax both the mind and body. For maximum stress relief, try to get at least 30 minutes of heart-pounding activity on most days. If it's easier to fit into your schedule, break up the activity into two or three shorter segments.

Make food choices that keep you going

Low blood sugar can make you feel anxious and irritable, while eating too much can make you lethargic. Healthy eating can help you get through stressful work days. By eating small but frequent meals, you can help your body maintain an even level of blood sugar, keep your energy up, stay focused, and avoid mood swings.

Drink alcohol in moderation and avoid nicotine

Alcohol temporarily reduces anxiety and worry, but too much can cause anxiety as it wears off. Drinking to relieve job stress may also eventually lead to alcohol abuse and dependence. Similarly, smoking when you are feeling stressed and overwhelmed may seem calming, but nicotine is a powerful stimulant – leading to higher, not lower, levels of anxiety.

Get enough sleep

Not only can stress and worry can cause insomnia, but a lack of sleep can leave you vulnerable to even more stress. When you are well-rested, it's much easier to keep your emotional balance, a key factor in coping with job and workplace stress. Try to improve the quality of your sleep by keeping a sleep schedule and aiming for 8 hours a night.

Get support

Close relationships are vital to helping you through times of stress so reach out to family and friends. Simply sharing your feelings face to face with another person can help relieve some of the stress. The other person doesn't have to ret to "fix" your problems; he or she just has to be a good listener. Accepting support is not a sign of weakness and it won't mean you are a burden to others. In fact, most friends will be flattered that you trust them enough to confide in them, and it will only strengthen your bond.

Tip 3: Reduce job stress by prioritizing and organizing

When job and workplace stress threatens to overwhelm you, there are simple steps you can take to regain control over yourself and the situation. Your newfound ability to maintain a sense of self-control in stressful situations will often be well-received by coworkers, managers, and subordinates alike, which can lead to better relationships at work. Here are some suggestions for reducing job stress by prioritizing and organizing your responsibilities.

Time management tips for reducing job stress

* Create a balanced schedule. Analyze your schedule, responsibilities, and daily tasks. All work and no play is a recipe for burnout. Try to find a balance between work and family life, social activities and solitary

pursuits, daily responsibilities and downtime.

* Don't over-commit yourself. Avoid scheduling things back-to-back or trying to fit too much into one day. All too often, we underestimate how long things will take. If you've got too much on your plate, distinguish between the "shoulds" and the "musts." Drop tasks that are not truly necessary to the bottom of the list or eliminate them entirely.

* Try to leave earlier in the morning. Even 10-15 minutes can make the difference between frantically rushing to your desk and having time to ease into your day. Don't add to your stress levels by running late.

* Plan regular breaks. Make sure to take short breaks throughout the day to take a walk or sit back and clear your mind. Also try to get away from your desk or work station for lunch. Stepping away from work to briefly relax and recharge will help you be more, not less, productive.

Task management tips for reducing job stress

* Prioritize tasks. Make a list of tasks you have to do, and tackle them in order of importance. Do the high-priority items first. If you have something particularly unpleasant to do, get it over with early. The rest of your day will be more pleasant as a result.

* Break projects into small steps. If a large project seems overwhelming, make a step-by-step plan. Focus on one manageable step at a time, rather than taking on everything at once.

* Delegate responsibility. You don't have to do it all yourself. If other people can take care of the task, why not let them? Let go of the desire to control or oversee every little step. You'll be letting go of unnecessary stress in the process.

* Be willing to compromise. When you ask someone to contribute differently to a task, revise a deadline, or change their behavior at work, be willing to do the same. Sometimes, if you can both bend a little, you'll be able to find a happy middle ground that reduces the stress levels for everyone.

Tip 4: Reduce job stress by improving emotional intelligence

Even if you are in a job where the environment has grown increasingly stressful, you can retain a large measure of self-control and self-confidence by understanding and practicing emotional intelligence. Emotional intelligence is the ability to manage and use your emotions in positive and constructive ways. When it comes to satisfaction and success at work, emotional intelligence matters just as much as intellectual ability. Emotional intelligence is about communicating with others in ways that draw people to you, overcome differences, repair wounded feelings, and defuse tension and stress.

Emotional intelligence in the workplace:

Emotional intelligence in the workplace has four major components:

- * Self-awareness – The ability to recognize your emotions and their impact while using gut feelings to guide your decisions.

- * Self-management – The ability to control your emotions and behavior and adapt to changing circumstances.

- * Social awareness – The ability to sense, understand, and react to other's emotions and feel comfortable socially.

- * Relationship management – The ability to inspire, influence, and connect to others and manage conflict.

The five key skills of emotional intelligence

There are five key skills that you need to master in order to raise your emotional intelligence and manage stress at work.

- * Realize when you are stressed, recognize your particular stress response, and become familiar with sensual cues that can rapidly calm and energize you. The best way to reduce stress quickly is through the senses: through sight, sound, smell, taste, and touch. But each person responds differently to sensory input, so you need to find things that are soothing to you.

* Stay connected to your internal emotional experience so you can appropriately manage your own emotions. Your moment-to-moment emotions influence your thoughts and actions, so pay attention to your feelings and factor them into your decision making at work. If you ignore your emotions you won't be able to fully understand your own motivations and needs, or to communicate effectively with others.

* Recognize and effectively use nonverbal cues and body language. In many cases, what we say is less important than how we say it or the other nonverbal signals we send out, such as eye contact, facial expression, tone of voice, posture, gesture and touch. Your nonverbal messages can either produce a sense of interest, trust, and desire for connection–or they can generate confusion, distrust, and stress. You also need to be able to accurately read and respond to the nonverbal cues that other people send you at work.

* Develop the capacity to meet challenges with humor. There is no better stress buster than a hearty laugh and nothing reduces stress quicker in the workplace than mutually shared humor. But, if the laugh is at someone else's expense, you may end up with more rather than less stress.

* Resolve conflict positively. Resolving conflict in healthy, constructive ways can strengthen trust between people and relieve workplace stress and tension. When handling emotionally-charged situations, stay focused in the present by disregarding old hurts and resentments, connect with your emotions, and hear both the words and the nonverbal cues being used. If a conflict can't be resolved, choose to end the argument, even if you still disagree.

Tip 5: Reduce job stress by breaking bad habits

Many of us make job stress worse with negative thoughts and behavior. If you can turn around these self-defeating habits, you'll find employer-imposed stress easier to handle.

* Resist perfectionism. No project, situation, or decision is ever perfect, so trying to attain perfection on everything will simply add unnecessary stress to your day. When you set unrealistic goals for yourself or try to do too much, you are setting yourself up to fall short. Aim to do your best, no one can ask for more than that.

* Clean up your act. If you are always running late, set your clocks and watches fast and give yourself extra time. If your desk is a mess, file and throw away the clutter; just knowing where everything is saves time and cuts stress. Make to-do lists and cross off items as you accomplish them. Plan your

day and stick to the schedule—you'll feel less overwhelmed.

* Flip your negative thinking. If you see the downside of every situation and interaction, you'll find yourself drained of energy and motivation. Try to think positively about your work, avoid negative-thinking co-workers, and pat yourself on the back about small accomplishments, even if no one else does.

* Don't try to control the uncontrollable. Many things at work are beyond our control—particularly the behavior of other people. Rather than stressing out over them, focus on the things you can control such as the way you choose to react to problems.

Four Ways to Dispel Stress

* Take time away. When stress is mounting at work, try to take a quick break and move away from the stressful situation. Take a stroll outside the workplace if possible, or spend a few minutes meditating in the break room. Physical movement or finding a quiet place to regain your balance can quickly reduce stress.

* Talk it over with someone. In some situations, simply sharing your thoughts and feelings with someone you trust can help reduce stress. Talking over a problem with someone who is both supportive and

empathetic can be a great way to let off steam and relieve stress.

* Connect with others at work. Developing friendships with some of your co-workers can help buffer you from the negative effects of stress. Remember to listen to them and offer support when they are in need as well.

* Look for humor in the situation. When used appropriately, humor is a great way to relieve stress in the workplace. When you or those around you start taking things too seriously, find a way to lighten the mood by sharing a joke or funny story.

Tip 6: Learn how managers or employers can reduce job stress

It's in a manager's best interest to keep stress levels in the workplace to a minimum. Managers can act as positive role models, especially in times of high stress, by following the tips outlined in this article. If a respected manager can remain calm in stressful work situations, it is much easier for his or her employees to also remain calm.

Additionally, there are a number of organizational changes that managers and employers can make to reduce workplace stress. These include:

Improve communication

* Share information with employees to reduce uncertainty about their jobs and futures.

* Clearly define employees' roles and responsibilities.

* Make communication friendly and efficient, not mean-spirited or petty.

Consult your employees

* Give workers opportunities to participate in decisions that affect their jobs.

* Consult employees about scheduling and work rules.

* Be sure the workload is suitable to employees' abilities and resources; avoid unrealistic deadlines.

* Show that individual workers are valued.

* Offer rewards and incentives.

* Praise good work performance, both verbally and officially, through schemes such as Employee of the Month.

* Provide opportunities for career development.

* Promote an "entrepreneurial" work climate that gives employees more control over their work.

Cultivate a friendly social climate

* Provide opportunities for social interaction among employees.

* Establish a zero-tolerance policy for harassment.

* Make management actions consistent with organizational values.

Preventing Burnout: Signs, Symptoms, Causes, and Coping Strategies

If constant stress has you feeling disillusioned, helpless, and completely worn out, you may be suffering from burnout. When you are burned out, problems seem insurmountable, everything looks bleak, and it's difficult to muster up the energy to care—let alone do something about your situation.

The unhappiness and detachment burnout causes can threaten your job, your relationships, and your health. But burnout can be healed. You can regain your balance by reassessing priorities, making time for yourself, and seeking support.

What is burnout?

Burnout is a state of emotional, mental, and physical exhaustion caused by excessive and prolonged stress. It occurs when you feel overwhelmed and unable to meet constant demands. As the stress continues, you begin to lose the interest or motivation that led you to take on a certain role in the first place.

Burnout reduces your productivity and saps your energy, leaving you feeling increasingly helpless, hopeless, cynical, and resentful. Eventually, you may feel like you have nothing more to give.

Most of us have days when we feel bored, overloaded, or unappreciated; when the dozen balls we keep in the air are not noticed, let alone rewarded; when dragging ourselves out of bed requires the determination of Hercules. If you feel like this most of the time, however, you may have burnout.

You may be on the road to burnout if:

* Every day is a bad day.

* Caring about your work or home life seems like a total waste of energy.

* You're exhausted all the time.

* The majority of your day is spent on tasks you find either mind-numbingly dull or overwhelming.

* You feel like nothing you do makes a difference or is appreciated.

The negative effects of burnout spill over into every area of life—including your home and social life. Burnout can also cause long-term changes to your body that make you vulnerable to illnesses like colds and flu. Because of its many consequences, it's important to deal with burnout right away.

Dealing with Burnout: The "Three R" Approach

* Recognize – Watch for the warning signs of burnout

* Reverse – Undo the damage by managing stress and seeking support

* Resilience – Build your resilience to stress by taking care of your physical and emotional health

The difference between stress and burnout

Burnout may be the result of unrelenting stress, but it is not the same as too much stress. Stress, by and large, involves too much: too many pressures that demand too much of you physically and psychologically. Stressed people can still imagine, though, that if they can just get everything under control, they'll feel better.

Burnout, on the other hand, is about not enough. Being burned out means feeling empty, devoid of motivation, and beyond caring. People experiencing burnout often don't see any hope of positive change in their situations. If excessive stress is like drowning in responsibilities, burnout is being all dried up. While you are usually aware of being under a lot of stress, you don't always notice burnout when it happens.

Stress vs. Burnout

Stress:

- * Characterized by over engagement
- * Emotions are overreactive
- * Produces urgency and hyperactivity
- * Loss of energy
- * Leads to anxiety disorders
- * Primary damage is physical
- * May kill you prematurely

Burnout:

- * Characterized by disengagement

* Emotions are blunted
* Produces helplessness and hopelessness
* Loss of motivation, ideals, and hope
* Leads to detachment and depression
* Primary damage is emotional
* May make life seem not worth living

Source: Stress and Burnout in Ministry

Causes of burnout

In many cases, burnout stems from your job. But anyone who feels overworked and undervalued is at risk for burnout—from the hardworking office worker who hasn't had a vacation or a raise in two years to the frazzled stay-at-home mom struggling with the heavy responsibility of taking care of three kids, the housework, and her aging father.

But burnout is not caused solely by stressful work or too many responsibilities. Other factors contribute to burnout, including your lifestyle and certain personality traits. What you do in your downtime and how you look at the world can play just as big of a role in causing burnout as work or home demands.

Work-related causes of burnout

* Feeling like you have little or no control over your work

* Lack of recognition or rewards for good work

* Unclear or overly demanding job expectations

* Doing work that's monotonous or unchallenging

* Working in a chaotic or high-pressure environment

Lifestyle causes of burnout

* Working too much, without enough time for relaxing and socializing

* Being expected to be too many things to too many people

* Taking on too many responsibilities, without enough help from others

* Not getting enough sleep

* Lack of close, supportive relationships

Personality traits can contribute to burnout

* Perfectionistic tendencies; nothing is ever good enough

* Pessimistic view of yourself and the world

* The need to be in control; reluctance to delegate to others

* High-achieving, Type A personality

Warning signs and symptoms of burnout

Burnout is a gradual process that occurs over an extended period of time. It doesn't happen overnight, but it can creep up on you if you are not paying attention to the warning signals. The signs and symptoms of burnout are subtle at first, but they get worse and worse as time goes on.

Think of the early symptoms of burnout as warning signs or red flags that something is wrong that needs to be addressed. If you pay attention to these early warning signs, you can prevent a major breakdown. If you ignore them, you'll eventually burn out.

Physical signs and symptoms of burnout

* Feeling tired and drained most of the time

* Lowered immunity, feeling sick a lot

* Frequent headaches, back pain, muscle aches

* Change in appetite or sleep habits

Emotional signs and symptoms of burnout

* Sense of failure and self-doubt

* Feeling helpless, trapped, and defeated

* Detachment, feeling alone in the world

* Loss of motivation

* Increasingly cynical and negative outlook

* Decreased satisfaction and sense of accomplishment

Behavioral signs and symptoms of burnout

* Withdrawing from responsibilities

* Isolating yourself from others

* Procrastinating, taking longer to get things done

* Using food, drugs, or alcohol to cope

* Taking out your frustrations on others

* Skipping work or coming in late and leaving early

Preventing burnout

If you recognize the warning signs of impending burnout in yourself, remember that it will only get worse if you leave it alone. But if you take steps to get your life back into balance, you can prevent burnout from becoming a full-blown breakdown.

Burnout prevention tips

* Start the day with a relaxing ritual. Rather than jumping out of bed as soon as you wake up, spend at least fifteen minutes meditating, writing in your journal, doing gentle stretches, or reading something that inspires you.

* Adopt healthy eating, exercising, and sleeping habits. When you eat right, engage in regular physical activity, and get plenty of rest, you have the energy and resilience to deal with life's hassles and demands.

* Set boundaries. Don't overextend yourself. Learn how to say "no" to requests on your time. If you find this difficult, remind yourself that saying "no" allows you to say "yes" to the things that you truly want to do.

* Take a daily break from technology. Set a time each day when you completely

disconnect. Put away your laptop, turn off your phone, and stop checking email.

* Nourish your creative side. Creativity is a powerful antidote to burnout. Try something new, start a fun project, or resume a favorite hobby. Choose activities that have nothing to do with work.

* Learn how to manage stress. When you are on the road to burnout, you may feel helpless. But you have a lot more control over stress than you may think. Learning how to manage stress can help you regain your balance.

Recovering from burnout

Sometimes it's too late to prevent burnout—you're already past the breaking point. If that's the case, it's important to take your burnout very seriously. Trying to push through the exhaustion and continue as you have been will only cause further emotional and physical damage.

While the tips for preventing burnout are still helpful at this stage, recovery requires additional steps.

Burnout recovery strategy #1: Slow down

When you've reached the end stage of burnout, adjusting your attitude or looking after your health is not going to solve the problem. You need to force yourself to slow down or take a break. Cut back whatever commitments and activities you can. Give yourself time to rest, reflect, and heal.

Burnout recovery strategy #2: Get support

When you are burned out, the natural tendency is to protect what little energy you have left by isolating yourself. But your friends and family are more important than ever during difficult times. Turn to your loved ones for support. Simply sharing your feelings with another person can relieve some of the stress. The other person doesn't have to ret to "fix" your problems; he or she just has to be a good listener. Opening up won't make you a burden to others. In fact, most friends will be flattered that you trust them enough to confide in them, and it will only strengthen your friendship.

Burnout recovery strategy #3: Reevaluate your goals and priorities

Burnout is an undeniable sign that something important in your life is not working. Take time to think about your hopes, goals, and dreams. Are you neglecting something that is truly important to you? Burnout can be an opportunity to rediscover what really makes you happy and to change course accordingly.

Recovering from burnout: Acknowledge your losses

Burnout brings with it many losses, which can often go unrecognized. Unrecognized losses trap a lot of your energy. It takes a tremendous amount of emotional control to keep yourself from feeling the pain of these losses. When you recognize these losses and allow yourself to grieve them, you release that trapped energy and open yourself to healing. These may include the loss of:

* Idealism or dream with which you entered your career

* The role or identity that originally came with your job

* Physical and emotional energy

* Friends, fun, and sense of community

* Self-esteem and sense of control

* Joy, meaning and purpose that make work—and life—worthwhile

Source: Keeping the Fire by Ruth Luban

Coping with job burnout

The most effective way to combat job burnout is to quit doing what you are doing and do something else, whether that means changing jobs or changing careers. But if that is not an option for you, there are still things you can do to improve your situation, or at least your state of mind.

* Actively address problems. Take a proactive rather than a passive approach to issues in your workplace, including stress at work. You'll feel less helpless if you assert yourself and express your needs. If you don't have the authority or resources to solve the problem, talk to a superior.

* Clarify your job description. Ask your boss for an updated description of your job duties and responsibilities. Point out things you are expected to do that are not part of your job description and gain a little leverage by showing that you've been putting in work over and above the parameters of your job.

* Ask for new duties. If you've been doing the exact same work for a long time, ask to try something new: a different grade level, a different sales territory, a different machine.

* Take time off. If burnout seems inevitable, take a complete break from work. Go on vacation, use up your sick days, ask for a temporary leave-of-absence—anything to remove yourself from the situation. Use the time away to recharge your batteries and take perspective.

Job Loss & Unemployment Stress: Tips for Staying Positive During Your Job Search

It's normal to feel hurt, vulnerable, or angry after losing a job. The good news is that despite the stress of job loss and unemployment, there are many things you can do to take control of the situation and maintain your spirits.

You can get through this tough time by taking care of yourself, reaching out to others, and taking the opportunity to rethink your career goals and rediscover what truly makes you happy.

Losing a job is stressful

Our jobs are much more than just the way we make a living. They influence how we see ourselves, as well as the way others see us. Our jobs give us structure, purpose, and meaning. That's why job loss and unemployment is one of the most stressful things you can experience.

Beyond the loss of income, losing a job also comes with other major losses, some of which may be even more difficult to face:

* Loss of your professional identity

* Loss of self-esteem and self-confidence

* Loss of your daily routine

* Loss of purposeful activity

* Loss of your work-based social network

* Loss of your sense of security

Grief is normal after losing a job

Grief is a natural response to loss, and that includes the loss of a job. Losing your job takes forces you to make rapid changes. You may feel angry, hurt, panicked, rejected, and scared. What you need to know is that these emotions are normal. You have every right to be upset, so accept your feelings and go easy on yourself.

Also remember that many, if not most, successful people have experienced major failures in their careers. But they've turned those failures around by picking themselves up, learning from the experience, and trying again. When bad things happen to you—like experiencing unemployment—you can grow stronger and more resilient in the process of overcoming them.

Coping with job loss and unemployment stress tip 1: Face your feelings

Fear, depression, and anxiety will make it harder to get back on the job market, so it's important to actively deal with your feelings and find healthy ways to grieve. Acknowledging your feelings and challenging your negative thoughts will help you deal with the loss and move on.

* Surviving the emotional roller coaster of unemployment and job loss

* Talk to a trusted friend or family member about what you are going through. He or she doesn't have to offer solutions, just be a good listener. The simple act of sharing can often make you feel better.

* Write about your feelings. Express everything you feel about being laid off or unemployed, including things you wish you had said (or hadn't said) to your former boss. This is especially cathartic if your layoff or termination was handled in an insensitive way.

* Accept reality. While it's important to acknowledge how difficult job loss and unemployment can be, it's equally important to avoid wallowing. Rather than dwelling on your job loss—how unfair it is; how poorly it was handled; things you could have done to prevent it; how much better life would be if it hadn't happened—try to accept the situation. The sooner you do, the sooner you can get on with the next phase in your life.

* Don't beat yourself up. It's easy to start criticizing or blaming yourself when you've lost your job and are unemployed. But it's important to avoid putting yourself down. You'll need your self-confidence intact as you are looking for a new job. Challenge every negative thought that goes through your head. If you start to think, "I'm a loser," write down evidence to the contrary: "I lost my job because of the recession, not because I was bad at my job."

* Look for the silver lining. Losing a job is easier to accept if you can find the lesson in your loss. What can you learn from the experience? Maybe your job loss and unemployment has given you a chance to reflect on what you want out of life and rethink your career priorities. Maybe it's made you stronger. If you look, you are sure to find something of value.

Beware of pitfalls

* Taking refuge in your "cave" may provide temporary comfort, but is little help if your time spent there is not constructive. Surrounding yourself with positive, supportive family and friends may better help your self-esteem.

* Venting your anger and frustrations may only make you feel worse if you find yourself in the middle of a "pity party." There are people who actually enjoy misery and the misfortune of others.

    *   Drinking is at best a temporary relief, and for some people, can lead to a crippling addiction.

Source: The University of Georgia

Coping with job loss and unemployment stress tip 2: Reach out

Don't underestimate the importance of other people when you are faced with job loss and unemployment. Be proactive. Let people know that you lost your job and are looking for work.

Taking action will help you feel more in control of your situation—and you never know what opportunities will arise. Plus, the outpouring of support you receive may pleasantly surprise you. Simple words of sympathy and encouragement can be a huge boost in this difficult time.

Turn to people you trust for support

Share what you are going through with the people you love and trust. Ask for the support you need. Don't try to shoulder the stress of job loss and unemployment alone. Your natural reaction may be to withdraw out of embarrassment and shame or to resist asking for help out of pride. But avoid the tendency to isolate. You will only feel worse.

Join or start a job club

Other job seekers can be invaluable sources of encouragement, support, and job leads. You can tap into this resource by joining or starting a job club. Being around other job seekers can be energizing and motivating, and help keep you on track during your job search.

To find a job club in your area, check out:

* Your local public library

* College and university career centers

* Professional networking sites

* The classifieds or career section of the newspaper

* Resources & References section below for links

Stay connected through networking

The vast majority of job openings are never advertised; they are filled by word of mouth. That's why networking is the best way to find a job. Unfortunately, many job seekers are hesitant to take advantage of networking because they are afraid of being seen as pushy, annoying, or self-serving. But networking is not about using other people or aggressively promoting yourself—it's about building relationships. As you look for a new job, these relationships can provide much-needed feedback, advice, and support.

Networking is much easier than you think: Networking may sound intimidating or difficult—especially when it comes to finding a job or asking for help—but it doesn't have to be. Networking can be rewarding and fun, even if you are shy or you feel like you don't know many people.

Coping with job loss and unemployment stress tip 3: Involve your family

Unemployment affects the whole family, so keep the lines of communication open. Tell your family what's going on and involve them in major decisions. Keeping your job loss or your unemployment a secret will only make the situation worse. Working together as a family will help you survive and thrive, even in this difficult time.

* Keep your family in the loop. Tell them about your job search plans, let them know how you are spending your time, update them on promising developments, and let them know how they can support you while you are unemployed.

* Listen to their concerns. Your family members are worried about you, as well as their own stability and future. Give them a chance to talk about their concerns and offer suggestions regarding your job loss and unemployment.

* Make time for family fun. Set aside regular family fun time where you can enjoy each other's company, let off steam, and forget about your job loss and unemployment troubles. This will help the whole family stay positive.

Helping Children Cope with a Parent's Unemployment

Children may be deeply affected by a parent's unemployment. It is important for them to know what has happened and how it will affect the family. However, try not to overburden them with the responsibility of too many of the emotional or financial details.

* Keep an open dialogue with your children. Letting them know what is really going on is vital. Children have a way of imagining the worst when they write their own "scripts," so the facts can actually be far less devastating than what they envision.

* Make sure your children know it's not anybody's fault. Children may not understand about job loss and immediately think that you did something wrong to cause it. Or, they may feel that somehow they are responsible or financially burdensome. They need reassurance in these matters, regardless of their age.

* Children need to feel they are helping. They want to help and having them do something like taking a cut in allowance, deferring expensive purchases, or getting an after-school job can make them feel as if they are part of the team.

Coping with job loss and unemployment stress tip 4: Take care of yourself

The stress of job loss and unemployment can take a toll on your health. Now more than ever, it's important to take care of yourself. That means looking after your emotional and physical needs and making stress management a priority.

Tips for managing unemployment stress:

* Maintain balance in your life. Don't let your job search consume you. Make time for fun, rest, and relaxation—whatever revitalizes you. Your job search will be more effective if you are mentally, emotionally, and physically at your best.

* Make time for regular exercise. Exercise can be a great outlet for stress and worry while you are unemployed and looking for work. It is also a powerful mood and energy booster. Aim for at least 30 minutes of exercise on most days of the week.

* Get plenty of sleep. Sleep has a huge influence on your mood and productivity. Make sure you are getting between 7 to 8 hours of sleep every night. It will help you keep your stress levels under control and maintain your focus throughout your job search.

* Practice relaxation techniques. Relaxation techniques such as deep breathing, meditation, and yoga are a powerful antidote to stress. They also boost your feelings of serenity and joy and teach you how to stay calm and collected in challenging situations—including job loss and unemployment.

Staying positive during a long job search

A long job search can wear on your attitude and outlook, especially if you are unemployed. If it's taking you longer than anticipated to find work, the following tips can help you stay focused and upbeat.

* Keep a regular daily routine. When you no longer have a job to report to every day, you can easily lose motivation. Treat your job search like a regular job, with a daily "start" and "end" time. Following a set schedule will help you be more efficient and productive while you are unemployed.

* Create a job search plan. Avoid getting overwhelmed by breaking big goals into small, manageable steps. Instead of trying to do everything at once, set priorities. If you are not having luck in your job search, take some time to rethink your goals.

* List your positives. Make a list of all the things you like about yourself, including skills, personality traits, accomplishments, and successes. Write down projects you are proud of, situations where you excelled, and things you are good at. Revisit this list often to remind yourself of your strengths.

* Volunteer. Unemployment can wear on your self-esteem and make you feel useless. Volunteering helps you maintain a sense of value and purpose. And helping others is an instantaneous mood booster. Volunteering can also provide career experience, social support, and networking opportunities.

* Focus on the things you can control. You can't control how quickly a potential

employer calls you back or whether or not they decide to hire you. Rather than wasting your precious energy on things that are out of your hands, turn your attention to things you can control during your unemployment, such as writing a great cover letter and resume tailored to the company you want to work for and setting up meetings with your networking contacts.

If you want further information, take a look at http://www.helpguide.org.

PART III:
ALTERNATIVE VISIONS

A FEW WORDS IN ADVANCE

Much of this book, draws on some of my difficult experiences.

My situation, like many of yours, was very traumatic, but it also very quickly shifted my outlook on many aspect of life, which provided me with some unique perspective on human behavior.

It presented me with questions that I might not otherwise considered, but because of SOM symptoms, those questions became central to my life and the focused on the exploration of myself.

If you have read the previous chapters, you already know that I went through every single specialist of eyes, brain, heart and soul ("soul" sounds better than mental health, right? and it is still accurate, since "Psychiatry" comes from the Ancient Greek words "soul" and "treatment").

Sometimes, there were simply no known paths to choose, and I had to try new ones.

I always choose the rational and scientific option, as long as science knows the answers to my questions.

In my opinion, a well-known scientific knowledge, is an unquestionable truth, which points toward the more coherent path to take.

The tricky situation is when science does not have the answer to –for example- how to deal with our condition.

It did not worth to mention every single experience, but in addition to those you read before, I had to deal with a gang of professionals wearing impeccably ironed medical white coats, who amidst a sea of uncertainties, were eager to offer -with an overdose of self-confidence- treatments that were actually experimental and that were only based on preliminary hypotheses, with unknown results.

It was so frustrating and I felt so powerless, that I had to go a step backwards to see the situation from another perspective.

I thought a lot about this and I concluded that when it comes to health and alternative medicine, the scientific ignorance is as reliable, as the alternative knowledge.

Meaning that a hidden professional uncertainty, is as vicious as an alternative conclusive affirmation.

The key words here are: "solutions" and "assumptions". This difference was everything at the moment I had to consider which approach I would be willing to explore.

I have never expected from a medical professional nothing but a scientifically tested SOLUTION, even if that solution was "you have to learn how to live with your eye".

On the contrary, when it came to alternative medicine, I have never expected nothing but an empirically experimented ASSUMPTION (not a cheap "as seen on TV" solutions).

"Medical assumptions" and "alternative solutions" were both taken as oxymoron, and both shared the same fate at the bottom my recycle bin.

In the previous chapters, I explained many of my experiences with several therapies that I have been trying along the way.

Said that, it is time to share with you, three additional approaches.

The difference of these lines in contrast with others (such acupuncture, homeopathy, etc.), is based that these ones relies exclusively on a paradigm shift, a change of mind set.

I know that this may sound as a new age stuff... accepted by some, criticized by many.

Unfortunately, people may relieve themselves of negative feelings, forget everyone, change lifestyle, meditate, pray, diet, exercise and take supplements, and yet, they are still suffering from what they wanted to get rid of.

The point with SOM, is that it was not caused by our thoughts, but it is just what it is. As far as it is known, you and I just choose the five winning numbers of the

SOM lotto drawing, and we got it, it was beyond our control.

One of the FAQ at the beginning of this book, was from a reader that asked me about if SOM was caused and could be healed just by the proper attitude, and if failed, you have only yourself to blame.

As a SOMer, and based on my empiric experience, I think that it is nonsense.

If it would be a matter of choice or attitude getting it, It should be a matter of choice or attitude getting rid of it, and it does not that way, right?

Believe me, I tried that one.

However, what I definitely found useful, is some technics to improve my self-awareness, the capacity for introspection, and questioning without judging about some things that could prompt SOM trough certain feeling.

Since stress is the major factor that triggers SOM symptoms, and generate a vicious cycle, in which in every loop stress gets more and more intense, perhaps some kind of thinking and some introspection, could help to get us out from that cycle.

This chapter is not intended to induce you to think positively, to see the glass as half-full even when it lies shattered on the floor.

CHAPTER 10.
POSITIVE ATTITUDE

Listening to your eye

During those sabbaticals, I recall the cover of a book I read many years ago, it was "You can heal your life" of Louise L. Hay.

She is a bestselling author, and an internationally known leader in the self-help field. Her key point is: "If we are willing to do the mental work, almost anything can be healed".

I remembered the key issue that was that our bodies communicate through physical maladies, letting us know when we are off or on the right track.

Hay says that all eye problems represent the inability to see the past, present or future clearly, or not liking what you see.

Far-sightedness is because of fear of the present, near-sightedness because of fear of the future.

Astigmatism is the fear of seeing the self.

Corrective affirmations such as 'I am safe in the here and now,' 'I create my own beautiful future', and 'I am willing to see my own beauty and magnificence,' allow the eyes and mind to live in harmony.

Daily life avoids us to listen the messages of our bodies, but she did an extensive list of maladies and the underlying messages.

If this assumption is correct, eyes related sufferings could be caused by fear of, not wanting to see what is going on in the family, fear of the present, fear of the future, looking at life through angry eyes and/or being angry at someone or something.

We –as an organic system- are designed to heal ourselves. All we need to do is to release ourselves from the emotional and physical obstacles.

All discomfort and suffering are just signals that a change is needed. Whether you blindly accept that SOM is incurable or not, you will be right.

The biggest mistake you can make is to blindly accept that SOM is incurable or unbeatable, your fear and mindset will avoid even the possibility of taking back the quality of life you deserve.

I am not able to confirm or deny this theory; however, I can say that it quite suited to my circumstances.

Your eye talks.

I do not care that much if it works or not. I mean, I do not care whether it is science or a new age good intentional suggestion. I just chose to believe it works, and it helped.

* * *

".... I never get infections. I do not get them. I do not get colds; I do not get flu, I do not get headaches, I do not get an upset stomach, and you know why? Cause I got a good strong immune system! And it gets a lot of practice! My immune system is equipped with the biological equivalent of fully automatic military assault rifles, with night vision and laser scopes. And we have recently acquired phosphorous grenades, cluster bombs and anti-personnel fragmentation mines." George Carlin. Fear of Germs

* * *

Even during a severe SOMday, I strove to think that it shall pass, recalling SOMless moments.

If such moments did occur, then they could repeat themselves, and eventually I could get gradually prolonged them until the point of make them steady.

Relapse episodes should be anchored deep in your mind reminding that no matter its intensity or frequency, recovery is certainly a possibility.

* * *

"Happiness is the harvest of a quiet eye." Austin O'Malley

* * *

Affirmations

You can change your perceptions and realities, your view of your world, both literally as well as metaphorically, and return to a natural state of clarity of vision.

Doctor Martin Brofman offers some affirmations you can use (Choose one each day and repeat it to yourself that day. From time to time, read the list to yourself):

* My vision is improving now.

* I choose clarity.

* I know what clarity is, and I experience it more and more each day.

* I remember clarity, and I am returning to clarity.

* I notice that I see more clearly every day.

* I know I can see clearly now.

* I know that my experiences lead me to clear vision.

* I accept new ways of thinking and seeing which are clearer for me.

* Acceptance and love lead to clarity.

* I accept what I see, and I see more clearly.

* It is easier and easier to see clearly.

* I am letting myself be real, and watching my vision clear.

* It is more and more comfortable to be myself, and see clearly.

*   My mind is reaching out and bringing to my awareness any information I need to experience clear vision.

*   I can have a clear vision today. I can see clearly today.

*   Every day, in every way, I am getting better and better.

*   I see more clearly when I am relaxed and centered.

*   I see clearly when I am here now.

*   Clarity exists here and now.

*   Clarity is my natural state.

*   Clarity is what is true for me.

*   I enjoy seeing clearly.

*   I see that everything is working perfectly.

*   I love when I see clearly.

*   Clarity is freedom, and being real.

*   I see more clearly now.

*   I see more clearly than I did before.

*   Today I choose to see the love.

*   When I do what I really want to do, something wonderful always happens.

*   I trust being real, and I see clearly.

*   I see clarity coming.

*   I can notice clear vision today.

*   As I clear my life, my vision clears.

* My vision is clearing now.

* I am free!

* My vision continues to clear as I adjust to my new state of consciousness.

* Instead of problems, I see solutions. I see the way things can work.

* Clearing my vision is easier than I thought.

* I know I can see clearly without eyeglasses.

* I agree with these statements.

* Affirmations always work!

What if we were wrong? What if SOM is not the cause but the effect? Would not you give a shot to that chance if it might help you to get rid of SOM?

Well, I did it. I had never been in therapy before but in search of answers I did not throw away any option. I had to get rid of some prejudgments, and I ventured to talk about what is going on with my eye.

As I get deeper in this subject, I realized it was connected with other emotional issues, not necessarily as the origin of my SOM, but positively as triggers.

I have found a correlation between some past and present emotional experiences and SOMdays.

Once understood it, I was able to manage the emotions in such a way that SOM got absolutely tamed, just as I meant it.

My Cockeyed Optimism comes not from being relentlessly cheerful or blindingly positive or eternally upbeat.

Cockeyed Optimism means that despite being fully aware of the problems and weaknesses; DESPITE all that and a hundred other things, I ALWAYS believe they have a great shot to find a way out and something better is waiting around the corner; always.

Do not ever thrown in the towel and stopped demanding your quality of life back. No matter what you think, no matter how you feel, the truth is you CAN do this.

You did nothing wrong as to deserve such a pain as SOM, neither I sustain that you can cure the SOM physiological root causes, just by the power of your attitude.

But stress management and your attitude, undeniably play a major role on your efforts to get rid of SOM symptoms.

CHAPTER 11.
VISION AS A METAPHOR

Eyesight is not just a physical process involving acuity. It is a multi-dimensional function affecting and affected by our emotional and mental state of Being, and linked to our personalities.

That is, each type of vision impairment correlates with specific personality types.

All nearsighted people have something in common in their personalities, and all farsighted people share a particular character trait, and all those with astigmatism are working with a similar issue in their lives.

All kinds of impaired vision represent stressed ways that a person interacts with their environment.

Some say that stress is responsible for all emotional and physical imbalances, and stress reflects how an individual interacts with his or her environment in a way which is not "at ease". Stress is stored in the physical body in a number of ways, including stress or tension in particular muscles.

We can say, then that physical tension is emotional or mental tension stored in the physical body, in the muscles.

Tension in particular muscles is related to particular emotions and mental states. In other words, where you feel the tension is related to why you feel the tension.

In the case of vision, different visual disorders have been identified with excessive tension in particular extra-ocular muscles (the muscles surrounding the eyeballs), and with particular emotional patterns.

To understand this process, let's look at how it works.

Surrounding each eyeball are six-eye muscles. We use these muscles to move our eyeballs in different directions, and for a while it was thought that this was their only function.

Then, it was discovered that these muscles are about one hundred times more powerful than they need to be to accomplish this, and since structure and function are related in the human body, it seemed evident that these muscles must have another function. They do.

The extra-ocular muscles also serve as part of the focusing mechanism for our eyesight, along with the lens. They cause the eyeballs to elongate or shorten, depending on what we are looking at, and what we are thinking or feeling. In this way, the eye operates more like a bellows camera, with variable focus, than a box camera with a fixed focal length.

Four muscles pull each eyeball straight back into the eye socket, shortening the eyeball.

Excessive tension on these muscles, called the Rectus muscles, creates a condition of farsightedness, and is experienced emotionally as tension in the consciousness, as coming out of one's Self, focusing on Image. It may be experienced as suppressed anger, or anger at one's self (guilt), or a feeling that in some way, the individual is not as important as other Beings.

Two muscles around each eyeball, the Oblique muscles, circle it like a belt, and when these muscles are tightened, they squeeze the eyeball, and it elongates.

Excessive tension on these muscles is related to nearsightedness, and this tension is experienced in consciousness as hiding within one's Self, retreating inward, as apprehension, fear, or non-trust as a perceptual filter, a sense of feeling threatened, not safe to be one's Self.

Uneven tensions on different muscles can create a condition of astigmatism, distortion of vision, by squeezing the eyeball unevenly in different directions so that the eyeball is pulled out of roundness.

This is experienced by the individual as a sense of being lost, as having uncertainty or confusion about their values, what they really want and/or what they really feel.

Values from the "outside" have been included "inside", in a way which is not natural, organic, or real for that individual, and the stress of this situation is experienced in the person's consciousness as well as in the eye muscles.

Impaired vision comes about at a time in people's lives when they are experiencing stress in relation to their environment, and do not see clearly at that time, both literally and figuratively.

When this goes on for an extended period of time or to an extreme of intensity, the eye muscles which hold these tensions may become temporarily "frozen", holding the eyeball in an out-of-focus condition.

Since the tensions in these muscles correspond with tensions in the person's consciousness, this also holds the individual in a particular state of consciousness.

These eye muscles can, however, be relaxed, and clear vision restored, using relaxation techniques and Hatha Yoga eye exercises (similar to what optometrists call "mobility training.").

When the proper "tone" is restored to the eye muscles, the eyeballs are able to resume their natural shape, and clear vision can return.

Tensions are released in the person's body, and consciousness as well, and there is a return to an easier, clearer, more natural (for that person) way of Being.

The natural state of our vision is clear, and returning to clarity is related to returning to balance, and really being ourselves.

Since vision is a metaphor for the way we see the world, and related to personality, once the elements of a person's experience that relate to their impaired vision are identified, they can be released, and clear vision can be restored.

Rather than being at the effect of perceptions we know to be distortions, we can decide to be at the cause, to consciously align with and choose those perceptions we know to be really true for us, and which will be more successful for us in our interactions, more in keeping with who we really are.

When we release the excessive tensions in our consciousness, the tensions are then released from the eye muscles from the inside, and the eyeball returns to its natural shape, and clear vision returns.

Naturally, since each type of vision impairment corresponds to a particular personality type, a change in personality may be expected to reflect the change in outer vision.

The "new" Being will have the same Essence of Being, yet with a different way of interacting with the environment, a different "dance," without what had been excessive tension for that individual. It will seem as though the individual had awakened from a very real-seeming dream, and things will make sense in a different way.

A perceptual filter will have been removed, a filter through which values had been determined, and without that filter, truer values will become evident.

The "new" Being may even have different tastes in food and/or clothing, and different personal habits, yet will feel more themselves, being who they really are. It will be a welcome transformation.

Approaches to vision improvement which have not considered the aspect of personality change has had only limited success. In cases where vision has been restored, the person involved has been through a transformative process and has, in fact, dropped a role, and become another Being, with another personality, more real, and with another way of seeing the world.

The degree of improvement and the rapidity of improvement has been connected with the willingness on the part of the individual, to accept the changes, to accept the new personality, to become the new Being, or rather, to become and live who they really are.

If we imagine that each of us is surrounded by a bubble of energy, our individual perceptual filters, we can see some metaphors. People who are nearsighted see what is close to them easier that they see what is far away.

They are more focused on what is in the bubble, and less on what is outside the bubble, preoccupied inside, not looking outside. Energy, the direction of attention, is moving inward, contracting, toward the inside, away from the outside.

Things must be held close to be seen clearly and comfortably. What one wants or feels is experienced as more important than what others want or feel.

One's orientation is toward Self, to an excess for that person. "I" is considered more important in some way than "YOU," and from the individual's point of view, "WE" does not seem to include "YOU" as an equal consideration.

An exceptional need for privacy may be experienced, a withdrawal from the world around them, a sense of being intimidated by their environment, a hiding inside.

The focus of thinking is forward, with fear or uncertainty as the emotional experience of that view. It is a preoccupation, keeping the individual from being totally present, in the here and now.

The degree to which this is experienced is a matter of individual balance, and related to the degree of nearsightedness.

Naturally, there may also be different compensations such as aggression to minimize the intimidation, or a forced extraversion to disguise the hiding within, but we are talking about the basis behind these outer actions.

With farsightedness, what is further away is seen more clearly than what is close. Farsighted people are more focused on what is outside the bubble and less on what is inside.

Energy is moving outward, expanding, away from what is inside, and holding away or moving against what is outside. Things must be held away to be seen clearly and comfortably.

What others want or feel is experienced as more important than one's own wants or feeling. One's orientation is toward others, away from Self, to an excess for that person. "YOU" is considered more important than "I," and from the individual's point of view "WE" does not seem to include "I" as an equal consideration.

While a nearsighted person retreats in readily and easily, a farsighted person has difficulty doing this since their attention continues to be directed outward.

The person experiences more interest in other people's lives, and avoidance of looking at their own. One's image is emphasized, and identified with, and gains more importance to the individual than the essence, who the person really is.

The sense of anger that the person experiences is suppressed, so as not to offend others. The focus of thinking is toward the past, with anger and self-justification, or a sense of not having done the right thing, and is a preoccupation keeping the individual from being totally present.

Again, the degree to which this is true is a matter of individual balance, and the degree of farsightedness, and there may be outer compensatory behavior, such as exaggerated saintliness to hide the guilt, or extreme kindliness to cover the anger.

With astigmatism, the bubble is distorted, and uncertainty of wants or feelings is experienced, depending on whether the right eye, or the left eye, or both, is affected.

Metaphysically, the right eye (the Will Eye) represents seeing clearly what one wants, and the left eye (the Spirit Eye) represents seeing clearly what one feels. In left-handed people, the traits are reversed.

In a given situation, a person with astigmatism wants or feels what is true for them, considers it inappropriate, and changes it, and then believes the pretended change, no longer seeing clearly what was really wanted or felt.

The focus is more on what "should" be wanted or felt, rather than what is real for that person, and a sense of confusion about who they really are. Who would they be if they stopped pretending to be who they are not?

Combinations of visual disorders are related to combinations of the qualities that have been mentioned. Astigmatism may be experienced in combination with either nearsightedness or farsightedness.

Naturally, these qualities may be experienced by others without the visual disorders, but for those individuals with impaired vision, these traits mentioned are particularly strong.

Nearsightedness means seeing more clearly what is close. Farsightedness means seeing more clearly what is far.

While in some rare cases, one eye may be nearsighted and the other farsighted, both conditions may not exist within the same eye.

When a person sees neither near nor far, the condition is one of rigidity of the accommodation mechanism, reflecting rigidity of consciousness, and relaxation techniques and eye exercises can restore flexibility. As a result, the individual will also notice greater flexibility in their mental process.

We are Beings of energy, and energy is directed by our consciousness.

Ultimately, we have the capability of choosing the direction of the flow of energy depending on the situation, choosing not to be directed by past patterns of actions or perceptions, but rather changing those perceptions which we know to be less than accurate or optimal, with a willingness to see things as they are, rather than through a distorting filter.

The flow of energy between the inside and the outside of the bubble can be changed, as can the nature of the bubble itself, which is, in fact, the perceptual "filter" through which we perceive our environment.

A "stuck" filter predisposes us to particular patterns of interacting and perceiving. It is like a selective lens allowing through only those perceptions which agree with the basic beliefs we have chosen or accepted, and ignoring or discounting all others.

Since we act on the basis of the information that gets through to us, we are then predisposed to responding to our environment in a fixed way.

The selectivity of the lens is not the problem, though the distorting quality of the emotional filter is what must be released.

When we are clear and centered, the bubble is clear, and so are our interactions. When we are in the middle of a strong emotion, we are not centered, and our perceptions change.

Situations look different, and so we respond differently. The bubble is distorted with the emotional currents.

When the strong emotions of anger, fear, confusion, etc., are suppressed, as is the case with those who have impaired vision, the bubble is also distorted, but the distortion is not recognized.

The person has identified with the distorted view and believes that it represents truth, and who they really are. In fact, it is not who they are, but just who they seem to be when functioning with the distortion. They can release the distorting aspect of the lens, and of their perceptions and return to their true clear selves.

Nearsighted people can direct the energy outward by being more and more willing to be visible to trust that will be all right.

In a given situation or interaction, they can see themselves as others see them, in a sense to see themselves through the other person's eyes, so that they not only have the view from the inside looking out, but also from the outside looking in.

This will give them the opportunity to step outside themselves, and see things from another point of view, and with the additional information thus gained, to use it to optimize their interactions.

It is also important to treat the other person as they themselves would like to be treated if they were in the other person's place.

It is not necessary to agree with the other person's perceptions of them, but just have the willingness to see that that's how they are being seen, and that the other person's perceptions are as important to the other person as their own are to them. In fact, the other person's perceptions might be very useful to know about.

The idea is not feel threatened or intimidated by the environment in which the individual finds him/herself, but rather to focus more and more on letting themselves be themselves, and trusting that when they do what they really want to do, and let themselves be real, something wonderful always happens.

And since that process is so important for themselves, to recognize that the same process is important for the people around them, also that everyone is just getting better and better at being themselves.

From the nearsighted person's point of view, "WE" can really include "YOU" as equal to "I," and in fact, just another "I," just as important.

Farsighted people can direct the energy more inward by giving themselves the same consideration they give others.

The idea is not to stop considering others, but also to consider themselves. There can be a conscious process of allowing themselves to receive without guilt -not to take, but to receive- and to express wants and feelings, and let themselves have.

When receiving, there need not be the need to reciprocate, or to deny, but just to say, "Thank you," and accept unconditionally.

Focus on accepting not only things, but also ideas. Notice any of the ways you have been holding things, ideas, or people away, and allow them to come closer.

There can be more a focus on who they really are, in addition to their image. Image is important, but Essence must not be overlooked.

Outer appearance is not more important than true sentiment, and people do appreciate honesty in feelings.

Consideration must also extend to yourself. Expressing love need not involve sacrifice. It is not necessary to come out of your space to be loved and respected.

The role can be fun, but also remember the Being who is playing it, the person inside. From the farsighted person's point of view, "WE" can include "I" as equal to "YOU," and "I" can be seen as another "YOU," as well as separate and important in its own right.

Astigmatics can ask themselves, from time to time during their day, "What do I really want now? What do I really feel now? What is true for me? What is real for me? If I stop wanting to be what I am not, who would I be? If I stop living up to other people's standards, who would I be?" If I stop pretending to be the person I have been playing, what would I be doing differently?

The feeling may have been that the real person would not be accepted in the environment, by the environment in which the person finds himself or herself.

Then, find out whether the feeling is real, by discontinuing the role, and being you. Either you will discover that the feeling was a misperception, and the role was unnecessary, or that the feeling was real, in which case you would be able to migrate to an environment in which you can be yourself, and be accepted. Either way, the effect would be a greater sense of ease in being you.

There's a place in society for all of us, and if we let ourselves be real, there's a place we really fit in, where we are not only accepted, but also appreciated for who we are.

We do not have to pretend not seeing what is real for us. We can all allow ourselves to be more and more who we really are, to be more and more real.

You can find additional information about Sir Martin Brofman, his articles, books and the Brofman Foundation at **www.healer.ch**.

* * *

From my conversation with Martin Brofman, I learned that when SOM symptom began you had a sense of separation from someone close since it is a problem with the nerves.

If you are right-handed and if it is your right eye, chances are that SOM is related with an emotional situation with a male, possibly father, a boss or any authority figure.

If it is your left eye, it could be the same situation but with a female. If you are left handed, the polarity would be reversed.

The scientific rationale behind this is that the left hemisphere of the brain rules the analytical thinking, and it is associated with the masculine aspect of the individual, controlling the opposite side of the body.

At the same time, the creativity hemisphere is located on the right-brain which is associated to feminine imaginative and sensitive attributes, controlling the right half of the body,

In case the two eyes were not working together, the male eye and the female eye, that it might not have been a harmonious relationship between your parents and that you might have been dealing with a sense of isolation, feeling alone in your story.

As strange as it may sound –at certain extent- this resonated with me and gave me some clue about where I should dig in order to get to something relevant that may be affecting my eye.

CHAPTER 12.
CAN OUR EYES HEAL
NATURALLY?

I still remember my first pair of glasses. It was after my sixth birthday, and I was the only boy in my class wearing them.

I recall how self-conscious and set apart I felt. The optometrist had told me that keeping them on all the time would prevent the number from going up. But that did not happen.

Over the years, my vision deteriorated, and I was getting a new pair of glasses almost every 18 months!

Today, my eyesight is not anywhere close to satisfactory. I have always wondered if I could cure my eyes. However, no one around me seemed to know how to do that.

Some help materialized when I did a 10-day camp in my final year of school which had eye exercises that would improve my vision, but it required me to go through life without my glasses, something I was conditioned against.

For many years, I have been trying to free myself of my glasses. My eyes are too sensitive for contact lenses, and laser surgery has had too many glitches to be considered safe.

The only option left is to enable them to heal naturally.

The allopathic viewpoint is discouraging. It views eye disorders as incurable, sees the eye as less than perfect and in need of crutches such as artificial lenses, which allow you to see well with your visual defect.

You are, therefore, stuck on this level of defective vision. Whenever your eyes try to function normally, your vision will be blurred. Now you can see well only when your eyes malfunction, and the visual defect becomes permanent.

But is this view the gospel truth?

I realized that all body parts have the ability to heal themselves.

I recalled the camp I had attended. I clearly remembered two directives: Let your eyes soak in the sun, and do as much as you can without glasses. And I started following their advice.

Sunning your eyes is best done early morning before 8 am. I try and use my eyes, in their natural form, as far as possible.

Only while on the roads, reading or on the computer I use my glasses. I found my eyes remain much more relaxed during the day, and that I do not need glasses for so many things.

Have you noticed that without glasses colors appear much brighter and objects much bigger? Yes, my spectacles power has not decreased but it has not increased either. And as the information given below proves, there is hope for me. Perfect eyesight may still be mine.

The myopic eye Vision disorders.

Some of the common eye disorders are myopia or short-sightedness, where the person struggles to see distant objects, hyperopia or far-sightedness where there is difficulty in seeing near objects.

Astigmatism causes blurred vision because the light focuses on two points of the retina instead of one.

Presbyopia is when a person has blurred vision at normal reading distance, and a tendency to hold reading material at arm's length. The macula is a small circular arc in the center of the retina, giving us our central and sharpest vision. In macular degeneration, people start losing that central vision and start seeing a black spot in its place.

The vision of the eye is not constant or fixed, it varies as per the emotions of a person, the external environment, stress and light conditions.

You can see better after a relaxing nap than at the end of a tiring routine.

Natural light is better than artificial light for reading and other demanding activity.

Bates Method

W. H. Bates, an American physician, developed a method to improve eyesight by healing the eyes.

His theory is that eye disorders are caused by stress. When this stress is removed, the eye returns to its natural healthy state.

The Bates Method is well known and his book, Perfect Sight Without Glasses, is very popular.

An optometrist's vision chart a very important technique in his method is palming. This is a practice in which the hands are used to softly cover the eyes.

The cheekbones rest on the heels of the hands and the fingers cross above the eyes, with the eyes resting softly on the palms. The hands shut out all light. The complete darkness enables the eyes to relax completely. Rubbing your palms together before palming is also very effective.

Blinking is another technique to relax the eyes. Blink fast and then blink hard, squeezing the eyelids together.

This lubricates the eyes and allows them a mini-rest. Splashing closed eyes with cold water also relaxes the eyes tremendously.

Central fixation is simply an awareness of seeing best in the center of our field of vision while at the same time remaining aware of our peripheral vision.

Bates' most important technique to improve eyesight is to carry on daily activities without glasses.

This technique allows the eyes to change back to their original perfect state. However, since this is not an instant step, it needs to be consciously done over time.

Yogic eye exercises

Yoga exercises for improving eyesight deal with eye movement.

1. Move the eyes to their uppermost position without moving the head, and then to their lowermost position.

2. Move the eyes to the left and then to the right in a horizontal direction.

3. Move the eyes diagonally from the top left corner to the bottom right corner; and then move them from the top right corner to bottom left corner.

4. Move the eyes in a clockwise and anticlockwise manner.

5. Stretch out your hands in front of you at eye level and focus on your thumbs.

6. Then slowly move the left hand to the left side and let the eyes follow it.

7. Repeat this with the right arm.

8. Then simultaneously move both arms outward and let the eyes follow them until they are out of sight. Repeat these exercises 10 times a day.

9. Focus on the thumb of your outstretched hand, then focus on an object more distant in the background.

10. Keep shifting the focus between the two to exercise the eye muscles.

11. Stand upright with your feet about one foot apart, and gently sway sideways like a pendulum.

Breathing is very important too; the eyes require a lot of oxygen for proper functioning.

Each one will take his own time to heal as it depends more on psychological factors than on physical ones.

Acupressure

The acupressure points for improving eyesight are the bony structure around the eyes, the eye sockets.

Pressure on these points helps the eye adjust and focus and makes you feel better instantly.

CHAPTER 13.
EXPLORING THE MIND/BODY
CONNECTION TO VISION

More than half of the people in the United States need glasses or contacts to see clearly, the other half expects that as they get older, they will, too.

Even though poor vision is the largest health-related epidemic affecting Americans today, even though younger and younger children need glasses and even though more middle-age people need bifocals and reading glasses, nearly everyone thinks that it is all perfectly normal and acceptable.

Poor vision is, quite simply, the problem that nobody wants to see.

Yet, doctors and researchers are at a loss to explain its exact cause. Although some still cling to the old belief that vision problems are inherited research dispels this myth: only 3 people out of every 100 are actually born with vision problems.

A Revealing Connection

From a holistic point of view, not seeing clearly, means more than not being able to see across the desk, across the room or across the street.

Being nearsighted is an expression of how a person views and responds to the world. Being nearsighted is a way of seeing or not seeing that goes beyond being able to see the bottom line on the eye chart.

We understand this subconsciously, if not directly.

Take the movies, for example. When a screenwriter wants to portray a character who is timid, shy, or unsure of him or herself, invariably that character wears glasses. And we in the audience get the message that wearing glasses conveys.

Behavior and personality studies on nearsighted people have been done since the early 1900s. Richard Lanyon. Ph.D., of the Harvard Medical School, co-authored a journal article reviewing the many studies that clearly document the relationship between personality and vision.

Nearsighted people consistently test as being more introverted, shy and lacking in confidence than their clear-seeing counterparts.

Spiritual teachers also recognize this relationship. Louise Hay, author of the classic You Can Heal Your Life, suggests that nearsighted people have a fear of seeing their future and of not trusting what is ahead in their lives.

Seth Speaks author, Jane Roberts, notes that for many, nearsightedness was a physical manifestation of something that they did not want to see on an emotional, psychological and/or spiritual level.

I have spent the last thirty years teaching holistic vision care, working one-on-one with people and conducting hundreds of workshops and seminars.

My experience confirms this relationship between the inner and outer aspects of seeing. My experience also shows me that it is not only nearsightedness that has a mind/body connection: farsightedness, astigmatism, eye imbalances even some medical eye problems also do.

The eyes are more than a camera. And not seeing clearly means much more than only that the camera being out of focus.

Our eyes are also sensitive emotional receptors through which we relate to others. We express our feelings through our eyes. We can often tell what somebody is thinking by the "look" in their eyes. And, in many ways, how we feel tempers how and what we see.

All of us have been in situations where we see things we do not like or that have hurt us in some way. Perhaps we imagine, "If I pretend not to see it, it will disappear," or "I do not want to see this part of myself or what is going on around me." Pretending not to see or not to know is one coping strategy that may be a useful protection at certain times.

The difference is that those who do not see clearly have ingrained this response into their consciousness, most often in response to particularly stressful situations that occurred prior to needing glasses the first time.

Vision Transition Period

I had surveyed 583 people before they began using The Program for Better Vision, a vision improvement audio course I developed.

I found that 63% of them were able to remember at least one significant change that occurred in their life during the 12 to 18 month period before first noticing a limitation in their vision. I call this period the Vision Transition Period.

The changes they noticed fell into one or more of these three categories.

1. Personal: Changes in self-image usually (but not always) accompanied by physical changes during adolescence (reaching puberty) or during middle age (aging), or changes in the fundamental ways in which other people and life are perceived.

2. Emotional: Changes in significant relationships. (Parents' divorce, another child is born, or a loved one dies.)

3. Situational: Changes in the environment. (Moving to another town and having to make new friends or switching careers, homes or schools.)

Whatever the specific external changes may have been, they are merely a catalyst. The key is that the emotional response of not wanting to see or be seen, of pulling away or hiding from the world, develops first on the inner levels before it manifests physically.

For the healing of vision to occur, it is necessary to release the habitual, inner barriers to seeing that first developed during the Vision Transition Period.

Notes one woman, Ruth G., after using The Program for Better Vision, "I found that I was intentionally blurring people once they came into seeing range...

This observation has carried the process to new areas and probed the deeper question of why I have hidden behind blurred vision."

One middle-aged stockbroker, Ralph P., who had been unable to see anything without his reading glasses, looked back at his Vision Transition Period -a time when he was losing money in the stock market.

He recalled that he had finally reached the point where he was afraid to look at the stock tables for "fear of seeing" how much he had lost that day.

The tables had become the "proof" that he was a failure and he did not want to see this image of himself as "being a failure."

As he let go of that false image, he saw himself as much more than his temporary successes or failures. Very soon, his vision returned to normal and, for the first time in five years, he began to read and work without glasses.

Not seeing clearly is, at least to some degree, an expression of one or more of the following inner decisions:

An emotional decision that we do not want to see some aspect of our self, our life, or our relationship with others.

A desire to pull away or hide from the parts of the world that we find either threatening, confusing or overwhelming.

Negative messages and beliefs that we may have absorbed about seeing. For example, a young child who sees her mother upset and is told, "Nothing's the matter" might learn the subconscious message "I can't trust what I see" or "It is not okay to see the truth of what is going on."

A shutting down of one's intuition or perceptiveness, which also limits our ability to sense what lays ahead in our lives.

The Total Picture

Glasses and contacts only deal with the symptoms of not seeing clearly. Using them does not address any of the underlying factors that may have led to their need in the first place.

They do not change the underlying patterns that caused the problem in the first place.

I have witnessed many powerful healings as people explore and release their inner barriers to seeing and being seen.

As people move beyond their habitual way of seeing, something extraordinary emerges an expanded view of who they are and of the deeper potential that lies within.

Along with this inner clarity comes the outer clarity: people improve their eyesight, reduce the strength of their prescriptions or discard their glasses and lenses altogether.

This inner healing is a crucial element. That's why I have found that people who only do eye exercises can be frustrated by their lack of improvement.

Along with releasing the inner barriers to seeing, the other elements of a comprehensive approach to better vision are re-training the brain and eyes to work together properly, reducing stress in the visual system and supplying the visual system with the proper nutrients and supplements.

Better vision means seeing the world in the clearest, most relaxed, easiest and most efficient way possible. Better vision also means having a positive image of yourself, a clear sense of purpose and emotional clarity.

* * *

The following is one in an ongoing series of columns entitled Your Eyesight and You: A Total Mind/Body Understanding of Vision by Martin Sussman.

Martin Sussman, an internationally known expert in holistic vision care, is the author of five books, audio courses and DVDs, including the #1 best-selling The Program for Better Vision and the Read Without Glasses Method (for middle-age sight). He is the founder and president of the Cambridge Institute for Better Vision, which he established in 1977. He can be reached at marty@bettervision.com. Information about his approach to vision improvement that is more than eye exercises can be found at www.bettervision.com.

PART IV:
LOOKING BACK

CHAPTER 14.
TWELVE MONTHS LATER...

I have been taking notes about my SOM experience for several years until 2013, when I decided to get them all together, and share it as a book.

Now, it is going to be an year since the first edition, and I can tell you: last year saw many changes that, challenged everything I wrote then.

I thought that since I had overcame SOM, everything would be better, but I had to face very tough times again.

Definitely, the major issue was that I -out of the blue- found myself unemployed. I had to face that, and seven endless months of job searching.

Everything about SOM was put to the test, which – although awful- brought a unique chance to prove under extreme conditions, if what I wrote was right (and if I had what it takes to deal with it, keeping me SOMfree). It was kind of a strength test.

So, once again, I put special attention to the experience, just as I used to do in the past, documenting everything.

Knowledge does not came from external sources. The only reliable way to gain any knowledge about how SOM works is trough observation, experimentation, and testing your guesses against evidence and results.

In retrospect, I think that playing the role of the observer instead of the victim, helped me to look at the situation with some degree of detachment, which let me focus on keeping SOM manageable.

I proved that SOM was far from being the center of my life as it used to be, that it surely can be tamed, and it positively could be of use.

If you know and want to listen, you can see in advance SOM symptoms coming, and you can learn to read them, as an indication to take preventive or corrective measures.

I enhanced the capacity to "feel" SOM coming before any symptoms could be noticeable, inferring in consequence -and with a significant accuracy- the causes.

This is like an earthquake warning device, that detects earthquakes fast enough that a warning can be given, providing seconds to minutes to prepare.

When I felt symptoms imminent, I knew if I should move away from someone, keep my distance from somewhere or avoid something.

I learnt how to recognize when my stress levels are about to get out of control or there is some kind of unbalance.

The most dangerous thing about stress is how easily it can creep up on you –upsetting your "rebel eye". I knew –just to mention an example- when it was necessary to breath deeper and relax.

It may be quite obvious, but sometimes it is really difficult to consciously become aware that you are breathing rapidly or with difficulty, or keeping a rigid posture contracting and stiffening your muscles, especially those of your neck and shoulders… and is not until you feel the pain that you realize of it.

I can imagine what you are thinking right now. I can imagine you, in the midst of the fiery struggling against SOM, dealing with all the discouraging feelings that it brings, that this is nonsense, irrelevant, or perhaps that my condition is –in nature or degree- different than yours.

Well, it is not.

You see, some people try to find a meaning to SOM as if it would be something out there to be discovered, some kind of divine and universal command that forced us to suffer from it.

Some people may sincerely believe that the meaning of SOM is a punishment, others may believe that is sort of karma…

But meaning is something that we create. The meaning you grant to SOM, will condition the way you live and your chances to move forward.

I chose thinking that SOM is neither a punishment nor a blessing, but a simple fact, a challenge and eventually something that –hopefully- may be useful.

My chose, shaped the way I came to terms with SOM.

It is understandable, that the meaning I granted to SOM, and the approach I chose to hack it, may resonate with you, but maybe not so with others.

That is fine, since there is not a common ground, a universal solution or a unique rationalization for it.

At the end of the day, the only thing we can be sure, is a common understanding about what SOM is, and that it is a unquestionable pain the neck.

If you want to know the answer to "why", in other terms, what is true and what is false about the very justification –if any- of our common condition and the way to handle it, there is no better method than getting to know yourself.

What is truth? Truth is the recognition of the reality, your reality. The point here is that the necessary condition to leave SOM behind, is to know yourself better.

I would not have had the chance to get SOMfree up to this point, if I would keep searching just external factors somewhere "out there".

Once you recognize your own reality, you will be able to choose starting a battle against SOM or find a way to get along with it, either way is right as long as it is your choice.

Whatever option you may pick, the true meaning that counts is the one that let you make the most with the one life you have.

Get on and live your life as fully and as well as you can!

Disclaimer: Of course, you can skip everything and choose to give surgery a try, getting a Teflon pad into your skull to compress artery and vein at the nerve's exit from the midbrain.

Pharmaceutical industry:
so long and thanks for all the pills!

Concerning the medication, I never really like the idea or accept the fact that I needed it.

So I consented it, but with the commitment of my doctor that I will not become captive of it. I asked her to lead me in such a way I could drop it as soon as possible.

I did not find anything funny keeping so many colorful pills that in contrast, a bag of assorted M&M could have looked monochromatic.

I started taking up to six pills a day, and now: none.

I will always remember the day I discontinued the regular medication...

One day the medical doctor that used to treat me, told me: "OK, Simon, that's it. You made it. Take just one pill a day as a transition, and later on you'll be free from medication."

I was ecstatic, and the doctor continued: "How do you think you are going to be with just one pill?"

"I will be great –I reply- as long as that pill is the size of an apple pie!"

So far, SOM symptoms still remains restrained, and I fortunately can say, that I had no relapse or whatsoever.

CHAPTER 15.
HOW I SEE IT

"One eye sees, the other feels." Paul Klee

* * *

So, this was my journey along the funhouse tunnel, though it was not fun at all, indeed.

In retrospect, my SOM experience seems unreal, just like a bad dream.

Once in a while, there is something that all of a sudden prompts a memory of it, and I could not help but be in awe, of the resilient attitude that it is needed in order to go through it.

I sincerely do not suggest you to focus on destroying SOM or drilling down to the sources and triggers.

On the contrary, I urge you to figure out how you can make yourself less vulnerable, which is another way to say, that I suggest you to focus on getting you stronger, instead of beating SOM.

I tell you: once emerged, SOM keeps there. Can you get rid of its symptoms? Yes. And once done, you will understand that it was you that got stronger, not SOM that got weaker!

Overcoming does not mean to ignore or destroy something or someone, but to reduce its capacity to strike or beat you.

How to keep calm and keep on with your life?

Minimize SOM's influence in your daily life, which eventually, let symptoms gently vanish away, and in order to accomplish it, you have to believe and accepting as truth, that it is possible.

It just does not worth wasting time blaming people, relationships, circumstances or anything that could have hurt you (even if you are right).

Above all, do not blame yourself for nothing! Do not judge yourself, since there is no reason you got SOM.

From my humble experience I realized that understanding yourself is the best way to pull oneself out of the depths of SOM.

Focus and learn from your emotions and thoughts instead of cursing your eye (you could be shooting the messenger).

SOM symptoms may be like the brake warning light on your car. If its light is on, you know something happens, and you do not even dare to cut the wire to turn off its light, right?

Well, same with SOM. It could be used as the break warning light, try not to focus on it, but to understand what that warning means.

You can put a stop to your SOM as you know it. You can manage it, curve it and get it over and done, in such a way; it will not be a handicap anymore.

* * *

"The struggle against anguish only produces new forms of anguish." -- Simone Weil

* * *

You are able to leave those SOMdays behind. They could become just an anecdote, making room for the amazing things that are yet to come.

Could anything good come out of SOM?

Yes, sure... wait, let me think.

Alright, there are four good things that you may get after your journey:

1. Perhaps you may assert that your already know yourself, but after SOM, you get to really understand yourself. You will realize what you really need, what you really want and what you really love.

2. After a challenge like this, you certainly will get more resilient and self-confident.

3. SOM symptoms become a very subtle warning alert, is the way your body talks to you. You will be able to take it as something good (not a blessing, but at least something useful). Many

people do not get any warning notice that something is wrong with their health condition. If you want to listen, when SOM bells are ringing, you have the chance to take some action.

4. Eventually, you will be able to enjoy what SOM prevents, and you will value those things we used to take for granted.

But no matter what happen, and beyond anything else, please, learn by heart the ending message of this book…

"It is only with the heart that one can see rightly; what is essential is invisible to the eye." Antoine de Saint Exupéry. The Little Prince.

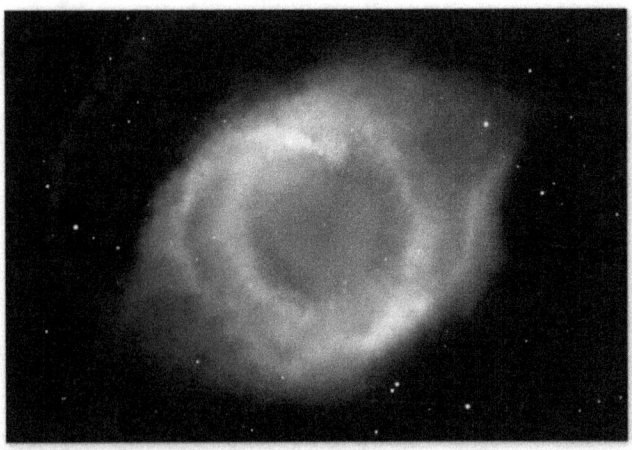

Picture 17: Eye of God. The Helix Nebula.

ABOUT THE AUTHOR

I am not going to write this section in the third-person, pretending that someone else wrote it, just to show-off.

The only appropriate acknowledgement as the author of this book is that I am a former SOMer.

I have no other merit that having went through the funhouse tunnel, doing my best to understand it, and eventually to share what I have learned.

Any additional comment would be superfluous.

I hope you have enjoyed this book; feel free to share your thoughts and comments as a review at Amazon.com. That will be my reward.

If you want to reach me, you can e-mail me at simonbeider@gmail.com.

The best,

Simon Beider

TABLE OF ILLUSTRATIONS

www.ingramcontent.com/pod-product-compliance
Lightning Source LLC
Chambersburg PA
CBHW051446170526
45166CB00001B/128